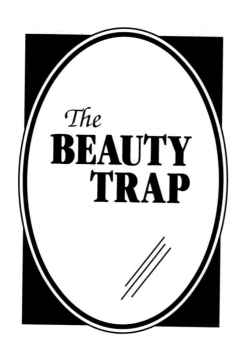

The
BEAUTY
TRAP

The BEAUTY TRAP

Elaine Landau

AN OPEN DOOR BOOK

New Discovery Books
New York

Maxwell Macmillan Canada
Toronto

Maxwell Macmillan International
New York Oxford Singapore Sydney

Design: Deborah Fillion

New Discovery Books
Macmillan Publishing Company
866 Third Avenue
New York, NY 10022

Maxwell Macmillan Canada, Inc.
1200 Eglinton Avenue East
Suite 200
Don Mills, Ontario M3C 3N1

Macmillan Publishing Company is part of the Maxwell Communication Group of Companies.

First Edition

Printed in the United States of America

10 9 8 7 6 5 4 3 2

Landau, Elaine.
    The beauty trap / by Elaine Landau. — 1st ed.
        p. cm.—(An Open door book)
    Includes bibliographical references and index.
    ISBN 0-02-751389-0
    1. Beauty, Personal—United States. 2. Women—United States—Psychology.
    3. Self-perception in women—United States. 4. Self-esteem in women—
    United States. I. Title. II. Series.
    HQ1220.U5L36 1994
    155.6'33—dc20   93-29641
    Summary: An examination of the various ways in which societal expectations and media images of women can lead to poor self-esteem and destructive behavior such as eating disorders. Contains discussions of cosmetic surgery and the new wave of feminism that is trying to break out of the beauty trap.

2/96 B&T $9.35

FOR DIANA LEIGH

CONTENTS

9 Introduction

15 Hear My Words #1: **Jenny Speaks**

19 Chapter 1: **The Importance of Being Pretty**

35 Hear My Words #2: **Krista Speaks**

39 Chapter 2: **Thin Is In**

65 Hear My Words #3: **Lynn Speaks**

73 Chapter 3: **The Magic Knife**

89 Hear My Words #4: **Molly Speaks**

93 Chapter 4: **Change?**

117 *Endnotes*

120 *For Further Reading*

121 *Organizations Concerned About the Status of Women*

126 *Index*

Introduction

**Before reading this book take time out
to ask yourself this question:**

If it were up to you,
which of the following options
would you choose for yourself?

OPTION A

PHYSICALLY:

You are breathtakingly beautiful. Your good looks rival those of a Miss America or Miss Universe, and you could easily win any beauty competition you entered. Ever since you were small, people have told you how lovely you are and suggested that you become an actress or model. You could walk along any beach in the world in a skimpy bikini and turn heads.

MENTALLY:

You are of average intelligence. You always do your best in school but rarely earn a grade higher than C. You tried to learn to play chess but it was too difficult to grasp so you gave up on it.

OPTION B

MENTALLY:

You are an intellectual genius. Your IQ is sky-high and you received 800 on both the verbal and math sections of the SAT. You're at the top of your class and people are always comparing you to Einstein. Your teachers predict that one day you'll bring home a Nobel Prize.

PHYSICALLY:

You've been called a plain-Jane, and although you aren't bad-looking, you've never dazzled anyone with your appearance.

If you selected Option A, you were not alone in your decision. It was the overwhelming choice of the many teenage girls to whom the question was posed. If it was your choice as well, ask yourself whether your thinking might have been somewhat shaped by societal expectations and pressures. Is life more fun for a "beauty" than a "brain"? Is it more important for a young girl to be sexually alluring than attentive in math and science classes?

This book explores these questions and others. It's about the beauty trap—a trap few American women can truthfully say they've entirely avoided. The beauty trap is actually a way of thinking that asserts that a woman's true value and desirability are essentially tied to the way she looks. Unfortunately, by accepting it and living their lives accordingly, women validate it.

Its entrenchment in our society has often come at a high cost. Women have developed dangerous eating disorders, undergone painful and expensive cosmetic surgery procedures, and endured uncomfortable beauty treatments just to look better. In the pages that follow, we'll explore the forces behind the beauty trap, its effect on women, and what some people are doing about it. If you've ever not gone to a beach or pool because you felt you looked too fat, worn uncomfortable shoes or clothing because you thought it improved your appearance, or had a bad day because you didn't like the way you looked—this book was written for you.

Author's Note

If you chose Option B, read this book anyway. The beauty trap is so pervasive in our society that no one—regardless of gender, age, or attitude—can completely avoid being touched by it in some way.

"Kill me, oh kill me! said the poor creature. . . . But what did he see reflected in the transparent water? He saw below him his own image; but he was no longer a clumsy dark gray bird, ugly and ungainly; he was himself a swan! . . . He thought of how he had been pursued and scorned, and now he heard them all say that he was the most beautiful of all beautiful birds. . . . I never dreamt of so much happiness when I was the Ugly Duckling!"

Hans Christian Andersen
"The Ugly Duckling"

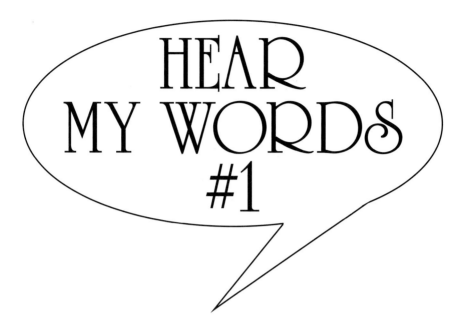

JENNY SPEAKS:

It was a steamy hot Saturday afternoon in July. My two girl-friends and I had just left the beach and were on our way home. We decided to walk along Ocean Avenue. It was the main drag in town and during the summer guys used to cruise it from midmorning until late at night. Some were local boys, but others were vacationing at the beach resort where my friends and I lived.

They [the boys] were always on Ocean Avenue. Rain or shine. They'd walk over there or drive through the strip in groups or alone. The boys came to look at girls in their bathing suits. Or at night to see the tanned, well-toned bod-

ies in halter tops and miniskirts. There was even an Ocean
Avenue dance club where girls wearing halters were admit-
ted free.

The girls, including my friends and I, knew where to
find the boys. And no one ever walked down Ocean
Avenue in the summertime unless she looked her best.
This involved a lot more work than you might think, since
many of us walked home along Ocean Avenue after coming off the beach. That meant you'd never leave for the
beach without a canvas bag containing your blow-dryer,
lipstick, blush, and whatever eye makeup you needed.
Then we'd spend from 30 to 40 minutes preparing for our
5- to 10-minute walk home.

My mother used to joke about it. She would say that
the girls walking down Ocean Avenue reminded her of
the elaborate dessert trays at fancy restaurants. There
would be rows of wonderfully decorated pastries to choose
from. I guess that in a way we were like those pastries. We
wanted to be desirable. To make the boys want us.

On that particular Saturday there weren't many boys
on the strip. No one whistled at us or yelled out, "Hi,
Gorgeous," or anything. I thought I might have changed
into my new bathing suit and sarong skirt for nothing.
But then something happened that the three of us weren't
prepared for. Butchie Langtree [last name changed] and a
bunch of his friends drove up and stopped their car.
Although none of us actually knew Butchie, we knew who

he was. He was a popular senior at school who had been dating the same cheerleader for over a year.

We were surprised when he pulled over. But Butchie only paused there for a moment. After quickly glancing at us he loudly announced: "Too fat, too thin, and way too ugly." A loud burst of laughter came from the car before it sped away.

We felt destroyed. Sometimes guys passed you on Ocean Avenue and didn't say anything, but it was unusual to get a mean crack like that. My girlfriends and I tried to ignore it. We pretended that we weren't hurt and just said that Butchie Langtree was a jerk.

But that wasn't how we felt inside. It was clear from the way my friends acted in the weeks that followed. Helene, the girl labeled too fat, went on a strict diet. It was funny because, while she wasn't skinny, Helene could hardly be considered overweight. Janice, who Butchie said was too thin, bought a push-up bra to make her bustline look fuller. She also began drinking milk shakes twice a day to put on some weight.

But what was I supposed to do? I was the ugly one. There wasn't a handy quick fix for me. I thought about having a nose job—I can't say it was the first time I'd thought about it, but my mother wouldn't hear of it.

I knew she was right. It was silly to consider going under a surgeon's knife because of what some boy I didn't even know said. A boy who probably just wanted to look cool in front of his friends. But Butchie's remark made me feel terrible and I wanted to do something to feel better, so even though my perm wasn't completely grown out, I permed my hair again. I felt it was the least I could do. I hoped it would make my nose look shorter and soften my features.

My mother thought I was ridiculous and kept saying that there are more important things than how you look. I guess I was too ashamed to tell her how I really felt about things. But the truth is that if a girl isn't pretty, she's nothing. Or worse yet, a joke. And I didn't want to be laughed at anymore.

CHAPTER 1

THE IMPORTANCE OF BEING PRETTY

"My aunt used to say, 'You're a pretty girl. You'll do well.'"[1]

Women are supposed to be beautiful. At times it may be an unstated requirement for acceptance and success in some areas of life. The message is so deeply woven into the fabric of our society that we often may not even be conscious of hearing it.

Children are introduced early on to societal values. Often these values come from childhood stories. Frequently these tales, which have been told for centuries, offer an idealized view of life. Good triumphs over evil, as do wise men over fools and virtue over sorcery.

The portrayal of women in fairy tales tends to be straightforward and unambiguous as well. Those who are kind and honest are beautiful and therefore worthy of love and esteem. Mean-spirited, evil women are usually characterized as ugly hags and witches. The underlying message is clear: A woman's exterior symbolizes what she is within. The essence of her existence and worth is intrinsically tied to her appearance.

Remember the tale of Sleeping Beauty. A king and queen have a baby girl and throw a magnificent christening party for the infant. The guests include the seven good fairies, who each bring the young princess a gift—one bestows the blessing of growing up to be "as fair as a rose."

Before the party's over, an uninvited fairy appears who is outraged at not being asked to the celebration. As you might expect, she's old and ugly and speaks in a shrill, piercing voice. The wicked fairy curses the small princess, promising that the girl will later die after pricking her finger on the spindle of a spinning wheel. Young readers see that this unattractive woman is sufficiently vindictive to plot the premeditated murder of a child. Although the remaining good fairy can't undo the curse, she amicably lightens it so that the princess merely falls into a deep, century-long sleep from which she can only be magically awakened by a prince's kiss.

The young princess grows up to be a beauty who is adored by both her parents and subjects. But as foretold, the teenage royal pricks her finger and falls into a seemingly endless slumber. Eventually the rescuing prince finds her and is so overcome by her beauty that he kisses her. At that moment she magically resumes her life. Unable to help herself for a century, the princess is only saved by her good looks.

Cinderella, another comely fairy-tale character, experiences a similar rescue scenario. After her father's death the girl's wicked stepmother and her two ugly stepsisters relegate the young woman to servant status. The others go off to the prince's ball, leaving Cinderella to sit among the fireplace ashes. However, her fairy godmother saves the day when she uses her magic wand to deck out Cinderella in a bejeweled gown and tiara as well as glass slippers. Although Cinderella is previously portrayed as having many desirable qualities, the prince magically falls in love with her as a result of her stunning beauty. In fact, Cinderella looks so beautiful at the ball that even her stepmother and stepsisters don't recognize her.

Although Cinderella flees the dance at the stroke of midnight, the prince manages to find her and make her his wife. Her spectacular beauty saves Cinderella from a life of servitude. Her fate seems remarkably similar to Sleeping Beauty's and the message to young children is the same. Little girls learn that being beautiful is the most important thing, while boys see that it's highly desirable to possess a great-looking woman.

Yeh-Shin, a Cinderella story from China, is quite similar to the European tale most American children grow up hearing, although it is thought to have originated in China more than 1,000 years earlier. Like Cinderella, Yeh-Shin is a "lovely" child "with skin as smooth as ivory and dark pools for eyes." And she is similarly mistreated by her stepmother, who is jealous of Yeh-Shin's beauty since her own daughter "was not pretty at all." Both girls want to go to a festival where young people often meet their future spouses. But Yeh-Shin's stepmother forbids her to attend as "she hoped to find a husband for her own daughter and did not want any man to see the beauteous Yeh-Shin first."

Yeh-Shin manages to go to the festival, where everyone is in awe of her good looks. The king later finds Yeh-Shin and is comparably enchanted by her beauty. As the story goes, "Her loveliness made her seem a heavenly being and the king suddenly knew in his heart that he found his true love."

Once again beauty equals value and desirability. It would be difficult for a female hearing these stories throughout her formative years not to make the obvious connection between good looks and a woman's worth.

The idealization of women is further reinforced through the toys children play with. Barbie dolls have been an American toy staple of little girls since they were first introduced in 1959. More than 500 million of these glamorous fashion dolls have been sold in 67 countries, and it's estimated that every two seconds somewhere a Barbie doll is purchased by or for a young girl.

As was noted by a financial analyst in *Forbes* magazine: "There's hardly a girl left on the continent who doesn't

own at least one Barbie. Mattel [the toy company manufacturing Barbie] has achieved a stunning 95% penetra-
tion with the fashion doll among U.S. girls age 3 to 11.
The average American girl had one Barbie in her toy chest
in the 1960's. Today she has seven."[2]

Barbie has also been successfully marketed to young
females abroad. The doll's overseas sales have amounted
to more than $700 million. The collapse of Communist
regimes in Eastern Europe in the early 1990s opened up
new potential Barbie markets as well.

Beautiful Barbie has long been an extremely salable
commodity. She's a leggy, adult-figured doll with a flow-
ing mane of hair and a voluptuous bustline. Barbie's supposed to be the perfectly formed, fashion-conscious
woman—everybody's dream girl. As one Barbie collector
explained the doll's appeal, "Little girls could project their
visions of their own futures onto Barbie."[3] Simply put,
Barbie's what's known in marketing as an "aspirational
doll"—children use this piece of polystyrene as a role
model.

But is Barbie potentially dangerous to a young girl's
self-image? What happens when the child turns into a
teenager and her body is no match for Barbie's plastic perfection? How does she feel when she falls short of what
she's grown up to believe is the ideal female? Marilyn
Motz, an associate professor at Ohio's Bowling Green State
University, feels that Barbie advances an unrealistic phys-

ical standard for girls to aspire to. If Barbie were human, her measurements would be 33-18-28—proportions that Motz cites as "almost not possible anatomically."

American Association of University Women head Susan Schuster further criticized Mattel in 1992 for creating a talking version of Barbie that said, among other things, "Math is tough." Some women felt that after over 30 years of silence, Barbie's first words merely underscored the doll's image as a brainless beauty with large breasts. If Barbie is an idol emulated by millions of little girls throughout the world, feminists wondered if she had to sound as dumb as she looked. Perhaps Susan Reverly, director of the women's studies program at Wellesley College, summed up Barbie's essence when she stated, "She's a bimbo. I don't want my daughter to think that becoming a woman means she has to look like Barbie."[4]

Ken Handler, the son of the couple who created Barbie, has also found fault with the doll, even though by his own admission the toy has made him a millionaire several times over. Handler has stressed that Barbie has "the wrong values." Instead of wearing glamorous swimwear, he feels Barbie "should care about more than going to the beach. . . . She should care about poverty and suffering in the world." He added, "I wish she would work in a soup kitchen, but then she wouldn't sell."[5]

Selling is what Barbie is all about, and girls throughout the country and the world appear to have been successfully sold on Barbie's glamorous good looks. As one Pennsylvania Barbie collector noted, "There is no doll in history that tells the story of a nation, its fashions and its fads, better than Barbie."[6]

Perhaps the closest human replicas we have of Barbie are the young women aspiring to be beauty queens. It's probably no coincidence that the first runner-up in a recent Miss Teenage America pageant cited collecting Barbies as her hobby. The Miss America pageant theme describes a girl "who took the place by storm," not with her intellect or personality but "with her all-American face and form." The song goes on to describe the contest winner as "your ideal"—she supposedly embodies what every American young woman should aspire to, and chief among her attributes is that she's exceedingly pretty.

Beauty pageants have survived through generations, and some people feel that's not a very encouraging sign. As in the fairy tales, pretty females are still being pitted against one another, hoping to be judged the fairest of them all. The competition begins at an early age. In fact, some small girls start their pageant training at about the same time they enter nursery school. These are the three- to six-year-old contestants in the Tiny Miss division of the Little Miss of America pageant.

Here small girls from throughout America come to Hollywood to participate in a rigorous five-day series of events that include swimsuit and party dress competitions.

Although the contestants are technically discouraged from wearing too much makeup, nearly all the pint-sized participants use lipstick, mascara, and blush. At a recent pageant, one little girl even wore a custom-made plastic cover-up for the space between her teeth.

Despite the girls' young ages a substantial amount of time, money, and energy is poured into preparing for the pageant. The girls' handmade dresses often cost somewhere between $400 and $600 each, and singing and dancing classes can annually amount to thousands of dollars. At these prices young contestants soon feel the pressure to be the prettiest for fear of disappointing their parents.

Being the best-looking of a group of beautiful children is a difficult assignment for any little girl, and when the girls' smiles, sparkling eyes, and jumps and backflips don't result in a crown, countless tearful faces may dot the pageant grounds. And winning isn't easy. At times mothers have charged that the judges favor blonds or that a girl without discernible dimples doesn't stand a chance.

But win or lose there's always another pageant, and many girls leave a contest with their hopes and dreams focused on the next event. Some do so to please a mother or father desirous of having a winning child. Others already believe that being beautiful is the most important goal a girl can achieve, and wish to be officially designated as lovely.

To an outsider, the pageant categories may seem inex-
haustible. The Little Miss of America pageant has five age-
based divisions ranging from Tiny Miss (3- to 6-year-olds)
to America's Miss (18- to 20-year-olds). The winners'
prizes at each level are designed to maximize the fantasy
surrounding an American beauty queen. Among other
prizes, a 3-year-old winner in the Tiny Miss division will
walk off with a suitably small mink jacket, a gold neck-
lace, $500 worth of Barbie accessories, and a $750 scholarship to modeling school (regardless of whether she
decides to become a brain surgeon or oceanographer).

Although many young contestants are extremely ded-
icated to winning, the level of seriousness attached to
beauty pageants intensifies with the participants' ages. In
a recent Miss America pageant Miss Oklahoma arrived
in Atlantic City with 17 wardrobe suitcases. One was
crammed with shoes. "I had 30 to 35 pairs," she recalled.
"They lined an entire wall in my hotel bedroom." Among
the gowns she brought for the pageant was a designer gar-
ment valued at $4,500. However, the aspiring beauty
queen gleefully remarked, "My family got a good deal on
it, and we only paid $3,700."[7]

While many beauty contestants claim to enter pageants
for the scholarship prize money, the actual costs involved
may, in fact, exceed their potential winnings. Prior to a
competition a young woman may have to invest in dic-
tion lessons, having her teeth bonded for a brighter smile,

sessions with a makeup artist and hairdresser, and exercise workouts at a health club. In some instances contestants also undergo painful and extensive plastic surgery, hoping to erase even minor facial and body flaws in order to enhance their chances of success.

On the final night of the pageant the stage will be filled with a glistening array of hopefuls, all looking their best. They send out an often detrimental message to the hundreds of thousands of young American women watching them on TV. Perhaps the overall effect was best summed up by a pageant critic who noted: "As the camera comes in on row upon row of smiling blondes, redheads, and brunettes, you compare your teeth to their teeth, your nose to their noses. They're beauty queens, after all, and they all have the look—that vibrant, leggy, flashy, confident look. They radiate something so clearly desirable in a young woman, so cheerfully and prettily, and girlishly American. Which brings you to your next thought. You're American too. . . . If your hair were pulled back and you lost ten pounds and had that glamorous makeup and that sequined swimsuit and those spikes—I mean, you hate spikes and sequins, but just if you wanted to—would it ever be possible that you could be in that lineup?"[8]

But perhaps the more important question is, should you want to be? Do those young women really look that way, or have they largely been polished to present an image designed to peddle beauty products? Since these women are esteemed as the essence of desirability, the advertising media have convinced us that the women represent the best of American womanhood. Yet as an observer of a recent Miss America pageant put it, "How many women do you know with a 22-inch waist who can twirl their batons while singing the national anthem without mussing their hair?"[9]

Much of the pageant glitz is actually based on illusion. On one occasion the public learned that a contestant's "perfect" figure was not what it seemed after a jealous competitor revealed that the young woman in question had stuffed her bra with toilet paper. Another year a fuss was made at the Miss America pageant following a contestant's admission that she'd sprayed her backside with adhesive glue to keep her swimsuit in place.

Would-be beauty queens have also wrapped themselves in cellophane to sweat off excess water weight, pushed their breasts together with surgical tape for a more voluptuous evening gown look, and worn specially structured swimsuits to improve their figures. Yet these are only minor deceptions compared to the significant plastic surgery and arduous weight reduction regimes some contestants undergo to transform themselves into pageant material.

Beauty pageants are big business. But to buy the products endorsed by beauty queens, the public first has to buy the fantasy behind the myth. Women have to believe that if they do whatever is necessary, regardless of the discomfort or cost involved, they'll come close to looking like a winning contestant. Comparably, men must be assured that dating or marrying a beauty queen is a measure of their success. As a result, young girls are left believing that a beautiful woman will forever be cherished by a modern-day prince. It's the Cinderella story of the nineties.

But do most beauty queens actually lead fantasy lives with fairy-tale endings? And do the rewards make the inherent expense and pain of their pursuit of glamour worthwhile? In reality beauty queens rarely enjoy the charmed existences we picture them as having. Ironically, many have even had to cope with tumultuous and scandal-ridden lives.

For example, one of the earliest Miss America contestants was later tried and acquitted in the shooting death of her jealous husband. Shortly thereafter, another Miss America ended her marriage in a highly publicized courtroom battle. During the trial the woman's maid testified that the former beauty queen sipped alcoholic beverages with her two-year-old child. To make matters worse, a locksmith who'd worked at the residence added that both the woman and her mother frequently entertained men at the house while her husband was away on business.

Miss America of 1937 didn't even show up to begin her reign. Instead, the morning after being crowned she sailed off to sea with a male companion. More recently a Miss America contestant was charged with drunken driving after running down a mailbox, while a former Miss Ohio pleaded guilty to a shoplifting charge that was eventually dropped.

Among the more publicized Miss America tragedies was Carolyn Suzanne Sapp's (Miss America 1992) experience of being beaten and terrorized by her boyfriend. Sapp met her professional football player boyfriend at a Just Say No to Drugs rally in Hawaii during her reign as Miss Kona Coffee, a title she held prior to becoming Miss America. The two fell in love and soon afterward became engaged.

However, their storybook romance darkened when Sapp's fiancé grew abusive after being cut from the football team he played for. One night while the couple was out walking, he became enraged and directed his anger at the beauty queen. He struck her and repeatedly kicked her after she fell to the ground. Although Sapp was not seriously injured, she was shaken by the violent actions of a man she thought she knew. Nevertheless, she took him back after he tearfully apologized and begged her forgiveness.

It seemed as if his blowup was just an isolated incident, until later that year when his fury was again unleashed after he was cut from a second ball team. Sapp was driving when her boyfriend tried to strangle her with her seat belt as well as push her from the moving car. The beauty queen fought for her life and managed to bring the vehicle to a stop in a nearby parking lot. Her boyfriend jumped out and was about to open the door to attack her from the driver's side when she quickly sped away.

Although the beauty queen ended her engagement, she decided that she and her former boyfriend could still be friends. Perhaps that's why she was especially vulnerable when he contacted her after being cut from a third football team. He called at three o'clock in the morning claiming to be drunk at a bar and in need of a ride. Sapp picked him up and brought him to a friend's house, where he was to spend the night. But when she got up to leave, he became infuriated.

Making it clear that he was still bitter about their breakup, he grabbed Sapp as she tried to go and threw her against the wall and onto the floor. He jumped on top of her and repeatedly slammed her body up and down. Then he took out a knife and pressed it against Sapp's face, threatening to kill her. Fortunately, she was saved when the man whose house her ex-boyfriend was staying at came in and pulled her attacker off her. The following day the beauty queen filed a restraining order in the Hawaii District Court against the man she had once loved and planned to marry. The abuse and their old relationship were finally over, but she'd been through a harrowing ordeal.

Ill-fated beauty queens are readily found outside the Miss America pageant as well. The Miss Universes of the world have endured their share of misfortune. Following her reign, Georgina Rizk, Miss Universe of 1971, was thought to have married a brilliant and handsome man. Unfortunately, her husband, Abu Hassan, turned out to be an infamous PLO terrorist. He was credited with masterminding the 1972 massacre of Israeli athletes at the Munich Olympic Games before being killed seven years later by a car bomb. Miss Universe of 1974, Amparo Munoz of Spain, became a controversial figure after developing a reputation for being temperamental and lacking self-control. Though out of the country at the time, in 1985 she was sentenced in absentia to a year in jail for hitting a film director and pulling his hair.

Undeniably, after stepping off the stage, beauty queens do not always lead beautiful lives. The guaranteed "happily ever after" ending is as unreal as the glamorous image pageants continue to project. Whether it's Miss America, Miss Universe, Miss Teenage America, Little Miss of America, or a host of others, beauty contests perpetuate a largely unattainable fantasy.

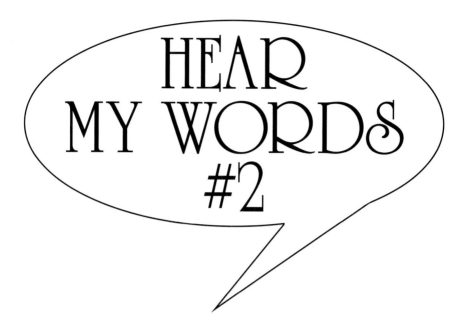

KRISTA SPEAKS:

When my parents split three years ago, my sister, Leah, went down south to live with my mother and I stayed up north with my father. I know it hurt my mom, but I had to do it. I told my mother that I didn't want to leave my friends and change schools, but that wasn't why. It was because of the weight thing.

My mother is really nuts when it comes to weight and appearance. She thinks there's nothing more important for a girl than looking good. My sister agrees with her, and the two of them have been on a lifelong diet. I love them both, but it's hard to be around Leah and Mom. I'm not fat, but I'm not a size 4 either, and they consider a girl who's size 12 unsightly.

Maybe I'd like to be thinner, but whenever I've taken off weight I've always put it back on within months. Before the divorce my father used to tell my mother to leave me alone but she'd tell him not to shield me from the truth. I guess to her the truth was that I was fat and not making the most of my looks.

I know that when you're thin people treat you differently. When my sister, mother, and I have gone shopping together, the salesladies are usually nicer to my sister than to me. They act as if she's a smart, slim girl who's in control of her life and somehow worthy of their admiration. Even though I think it's wrong to treat customers differently because of what they weigh, my mother and sister don't have a problem with it. They tell me that's just the way things are and suggest that I try to push myself away from the table.

It was like what happened after the talk show host Oprah Winfrey gained back most of the weight she lost. All three of us liked her show, and when Oprah went on the liquid fast diet and lost about 70 pounds, my mom said that she should be an inspiration to me. My mother even called up a clinic to find out if I could go on the fast, but they said I was too young and wasn't overweight enough.

So Mom said I should still follow Oprah's lead and go

on my own diet. But I thought Oprah was really great
after she regained the weight. Now she was finally able to
accept herself and stopped starving to please others. I
thought it must have taken a lot of courage to do what
was right for her while millions of TV viewers sat around
judging her.

My mother felt differently, though. She said that
Oprah's lack of self-control was disgraceful, and that she
had disappointed her fans. But Oprah hadn't disappointed
me. Instead, she strengthened my convictions and I was
glad that a celebrity had shown the world that being overweight is okay. It didn't have to stop you from being successful.

Sometimes with them being so far away, I miss my
mother and sister. But I don't miss the way they pressure
me to lose weight. That's not to say that my mother
doesn't have a long reach. She writes to me every week
and usually encloses some article about weight loss she's
clipped from a magazine or newspaper. It used to annoy
me, but I try not to get upset anymore. Most of the time
I don't even bother reading them.

Still, I was really upset a few months ago when we
were all together for my cousin's wedding. My mother
always says that a girl has to be thin to attract the right
kind of boy, but I've been going with someone great for
over a year and we're really happy. But when I brought
my boyfriend to the church with me for the ceremony, I

knew from the look on my mother's face that she didn't approve. Even though my boyfriend, Mike, is heavier than me, he's got this terrific teddy-bear quality and I've always been drawn to him. Apparently that didn't matter. When my mother got me alone at the reception, she sarcastically wondered aloud whether Mike was going to eat most of the wedding cake himself and said he was the kind of boy a fat girl ends up with.

I was even more hurt when I overheard her tell my aunt that Mike wasn't my steady boyfriend. There was no denying it. My mother was ashamed of Mike, and I knew that she was ashamed of me for weighing more than she thought I should and for being with someone like my boyfriend. And at those times I'm really glad I live with my father.

CHAPTER 2

THIN IS IN

"In spite of our efforts to shape, adorn, shrink, rejuvenate, and otherwise control them, we do not possess our bodies. We have long since relinquished them. In all of these efforts we are merely acting as executors of the will of others . . . who have let us know from childhood what a woman's body should be."[1]

In countless ways women of all ages are daily reminded of the importance of being thin. Underweight fashion models peer at us from magazines, billboards, and TV.

These exceedingly slender females appear to be naturally thin, but in reality many retain their slender forms through a rigid and often nearly debilitating diet and exercise regime.

However, thin wasn't always in. As demonstrated by the women portrayed by the famous painter Rubens, between the 16th and 19th centuries females who would be considered fat today were admired for their physical beauty. Nevertheless, after 1900 society began to increasingly equate thinness with physical attractiveness.

Part of the attitude shift can be attributed to thinness being perceived as a sign of wealth, sophistication, and upper-class status. As a sociologist put it: "Being thin is a kind of inconspicuous consumption that distinguishes the rich at a time when most poor people can more easily afford to be fat than thin. . . . For a man to have a thin woman on his arm is a sign of his own worth, and a woman increases her market value by being slender."[2]

The tie between thinness and beauty becomes obvious to children early on in life. It may be all right to be a chubby baby, but an overweight adolescent is regarded differently. Accordingly, Cabbage Patch babies are traded in for Barbies as little girls become immersed in what's expected of women.

An overweight girl will frequently be dealt with cruelly. She may not be admired and sought after by boys, and may be reluctant to shed her robe at the pool or beach. Depending on how heavy she becomes, she may even be treated as a freak or referred to by cruel names.

Although she may be trying to lose weight, until she successfully conforms to the norm, she'll often be treated with contempt. Her deviation from what's socially desirable and the price she's made to pay for it stand as constant reminders to other young girls.

Most females in our society would go to any lengths to avoid being fat. In a recent newspaper survey formerly heavy women who'd lost a substantial amount of weight through intestinal bypass surgery indicated that they would rather be blind, deaf, or have a leg amputated than resume their former size. The plight of overweight women was further underscored when Leslie Lambert, an editor at a popular woman's magazine, went undercover in a custom-made "fat suit" to expose what obese people actually face on a daily basis.

Lambert, a slender working mother of three, was fitted for her fat suit by Hollywood special effects artist Richard Tautkas, who designed the costumes for the Ringling Bros. and Barnum & Bailey Circus, the Star Wars road show, and a number of Broadway extravaganzas. Although the suit he created for Lambert was lightweight, it added 150 pounds in bulk to her slim frame, making her instantly obese.

Since Lambert's transformation involved only her appearance and not her mind or personality, she was amazed at the brutality she encountered during the week she became an undercover fat person. Apparently those around her felt comfortable ridiculing and insulting Lambert simply because they perceived her as an overweight female. After Lambert boarded a train from suburbia to go to work in the city, the other passengers deliberately avoided sitting near her to insure that they'd have ample room for themselves. Yet the fat-suited magazine editor found that she was hardly ignored. People looked up from their newspapers long enough to emphatically register their disapproval. Two women even made unflattering comments about her weight, speaking loudly enough to be overheard. Before long Lambert realized that people were going to judge and dismiss her solely on the basis of dress size.

Although a business lunch can be a relaxing breather during a busy workday, Leslie Lambert hardly enjoyed dining with colleagues in a swank uptown restaurant while wearing her fat suit. Due to the narrow space between tables Lambert had to squeeze through to reach her chair while other diners commented on her form. It was also difficult to enjoy a meal while seated in a chair designed with armrests that were obviously meant to encircle a smaller person.

Later that evening, while driving home from the train station, Lambert stopped at a red light across from a car with two teenage boys in it. She happened to glance across the lane in time to see the one in the passenger seat puff out his cheeks in a cruel imitation of her before he burst out laughing.

As long as she wore the fat suit, Lambert's days were filled with similar incidents, regardless of where she went or whom she was with. When she ordered food for her family at a take-out restaurant, a group of children referred to her as "the fat lady," while the adults with them obviously found the young people's assessment amusing. Lambert also reported feeling like a criminal when at a supermarket she reached for a package of candy she had promised her children.

However, if Lambert found purchasing food difficult, the blatant hostility toward her mushroomed when others saw her actually eating. Restaurant patrons both winced and giggled as she ordered a goat cheese salad and pasta with cream sauce, while passengers on the train ride home looked at her in disgust after she hungrily bit into a bagel.

But one of the worst incidents occurred when Leslie Lambert and a companion were seated at the back of a fashionable restaurant, despite the fact that Lambert had called in advance to request a more visible table near the restaurant's entrance. Two women at the next table looked at her in horror when the water glasses shook as Lambert accidentally rocked both tables getting into her seat. While she was in the ladies' room, one of the women asked her escort why he was with such a fat pig. He indignantly told them that she was his girlfriend, but the women looked at him in disbelief and insisted that he must be a hustler. When Lambert returned from the ladies' room after removing the fat suit, the two women were angry at having been tricked rather than embarrassed over how they'd acted.

While the outside world was often difficult to contend with as a fat person, Lambert soon realized that her family was not unaffected by society's overall disgust at obese people. After Lambert showed her before and after photos in her fat suit to her children and spouse, her husband reconsidered his plans to dine out with his wife while she wore her disguise. Her children asked her not to wear it when she picked them up at school. One of her young daughters felt that she looked scary, while Lambert's ten-year-old said that she didn't want people to stare or hurt her mother's feelings by ridiculing her.

However, Lambert sadly found that being fat can do more than hurt your feelings or cause you to question the value systems of those around you—in some instances it can cost you your livelihood. Leslie Lambert visited an office temp agency while wearing her fat suit, pretending to look for work. Supposedly, jobs were available, and with a master's degree in journalism and word processing skills, she was a more than qualified applicant. Yet Lambert encountered the same disdain at the employment agency

that she came up against in countless other ways throughout the week.

After seeing her, the employment counselor she had
an appointment with kept Lambert waiting for nearly half
an hour. When she finally spoke with him, she stressed
her credentials, as well as how much she needed a job.
Although the counselor promised to call Lambert soon,
as might be expected he never contacted her.

In the end the slim woman's week as an obese individual proved to be both depressing and eye-opening. As
she summarized her experience: "There's no denying that
on a minute-to-minute basis, I met with serious preju-
dice. . . . You know you're going to meet with a certain
amount of disapproval, but I was shocked at how much
hatred there is out there. People are really mean, and it's
acceptable. It's OK to be rude, nasty, and hateful to over-
sized people."[3]

Young women see that beauty is a highly valued commodity—one that a fat girl can never possess. Regardless
of how attractive her face, hair, or hands may be, she
always falls short of the mark and is therefore looked upon
disdainfully. Yet ironically, this pressure to be thin exists
in a society where eating and good food are highly prized
as well. No one is overweight in the commercials for fast-
food or pizza places, yet anyone habitually eating at these
establishments might soon gain weight.

As psychologist Wayne Anderson put it: "As a nation

we have become almost schizophrenic in our treatment of food. Our ads encourage people to eat, we have richness of choices, and the prices are cheap in comparison to other nations. We are a nation where becoming overweight is easy."[4]

The tremendous pressure for women to remain slender in a culture where eating is practically a national pastime has often been cited as a factor in the rampant increase of eating disorders such as anorexia nervosa and bulimia. According to Dr. Diane Mickley, president of the American Anorexia/Bulimia Association and director of the Wilkins Center for Eating Disorders in Greenwich, Connecticut: "The incidence of eating disorders skyrocketed after the big societal swing started with Twiggy [a very thin model] in the '60s. There's no question that the prevalence is much greater than it was 30 years ago."[5]

Victims of anorexia nervosa are frequently triggered by an excessive concern with weight, diet, and body shape, and starve themselves through prolonged fasting or a dramatic reduction in their daily food intake. This stringent dieting is frequently accompanied by excessive exercise, as well as the consumption of large doses of laxatives. The anorexic has a distorted view of her body and how she actually looks. While others may beg her to eat, she refuses, and regardless of how thin she becomes, she persists in believing that she's overweight.

A gaunt, dangerously underweight anorexic wearing a

bikini can stand in front of a mirror with her therapist and describe herself as obese and flabby. As the disorder continues, the telltale physical signs become evident. Anorexics often experience difficulty moving their bowels, and many stop menstruating. Their skin becomes excessively dry, while their hair appears dull and stringy.

As their weight continues to drop, a growth of fine hair known as lanugo will cover portions of their bodies. Without effective medical intervention they may eventually develop irregular heart rhythms. The anorexic's ongoing self-induced starvation frequently results in a loss of 25 percent or more of the woman's body weight. An estimated 6 to 10 percent of anorexics die as a result of the disorder.

Anorexics are not afraid of food—they fear becoming fat. And although they may refuse to eat, they are frequently preoccupied with thoughts of food. Often their obsession with weight becomes the focal point of their lives as they tend to withdraw from former friendships and their school or work performance falters.

Perhaps the following case best illustrates how anorexia nervosa can overpower and debilitate a young person's life.

Amy M.'s mother enrolled her in ballet class when she was just three, and by the time she was seven the young girl had her heart set on becoming a prima ballerina. Knowing that her goal required a great deal of commitment, Amy willingly gave up most other after-school activities to have time to practice as well as take additional dance classes. After a while Amy's only friends were the girls she danced with.

She also turned her bedroom into a true dancer's haven. Amy covered her walls with pictures of star ballerinas and stage scenes from various ballets. A pink satin toe shoe hung from each side of her full-length mirror and on all four of her bedposts. As Amy dressed for school each morning and waited for the bus, she'd practice a dance step or arm movement.

Yet despite her love for ballet, by the time Amy turned 12 she experienced an unanticipated problem. While she was certainly not overweight, she'd grown taller and had developed a more ample figure than most other girls in her class. Upset by a natural filling out of her breasts and hips, Amy felt that she might never have the svelte form characteristic of professional dancers. She hated the way her blossoming body made her look, and felt increasing self-conscious in dance class. These feelings intensified after she realized that she wasn't the only one aware of what was happening to her. Now the other girls and even her mother teased her about looking sexy in a leotard.

Amy didn't want to look sexy—she dreamed of being as slim as the great ballerinas and increasingly felt as if her body were betraying her. Perhaps the most painful moment occurred when she was rejected for a local production of "The Nutcracker." Amy felt certain that she was as talented as the girls selected but had looked too mature for the part.

A few weeks later Amy asked her family doctor for diet pills, but he insisted that she didn't need to diet. Yet despite her doctor's and parents' warnings Amy began limiting what she ate. When her mother noticed her skipping snacks and eating less at meals, Amy lied, assuring her mother that she was only trying to maintain her weight.

Nevertheless, Amy avoided food whenever possible. She made a habit of filling up on vegetables and passing on the meats, starches, and desserts. She'd also purposely try to be out of the house at dinnertime, and when her mother offered to fix her something to eat Amy would say that she'd already eaten at a friend's house. On days when it was impossible for her to get away and her parents insisted that she eat a balanced, nutritional meal, she'd force herself to vomit afterward.

Amy spent her lunch money on large quantities of sugarless gum, which soon became the mainstay of her diet. When her mother packed an ample lunch for her, she gave it to a homeless man who camped out near the school. Amy pursued dieting with the same rigor she'd put into dancing and was determined to let nothing stand in her way.

Within weeks the young dancer began to look thinner, and before long she weighed considerably less than she should have for her height and build. She knew there'd be problems if her parents knew what she was up to, so Amy did her best to hide it from them. She was careful not to let them see her in a leotard, which would have revealed her emaciated body. Instead of practicing at home, she began spending most of her spare time at the dance studio. She practiced more than ever—not so much to perfect her movements as to burn off the minimal calories she ingested. Amy also changed the way she dressed to further conceal her weight loss. She switched from miniskirts and form-fitting turtlenecks to baggy sweaters and loose-fitting layered outfits.

As time passed, it was evident that Amy had lost her perspective on dieting. Rather than allow herself more calories once she was thinner, she became increasingly rigid regarding her intake. When her aunt and uncle took her to her favorite Chinese restaurant for her birthday, Amy ordered shrimp in black bean sauce and only ate six black beans. Seeing her aunt's and uncle's distress, Amy told them that she'd eaten too much at lunch and couldn't take another bite. They insisted that Amy take home the meal to enjoy later, but their niece dropped the doggie bag into the trash can as soon as her relatives drove away.

By now Amy's entire life revolved around dieting. She felt pressured to hide the truth from her parents, and her Olympiclike exercise regime, self-induced vomiting, and restricted caloric intake often left her exhausted and depressed. When her friends seemed concerned about her weight loss, Amy stopped seeing them. She became socially withdrawn, convincing herself that her friends were jealous and didn't want her to be thin and get all the best dance roles. In time Amy became so preoccupied with dieting that her grades dropped along with her weight.

There's no telling how long Amy's masquerade would have continued if her mother hadn't accidentally walked in on her while she was dressing. Her mother was so shocked at the sight of her daughter, who was now just skin and bones, that she shouted, "My God, what's happened to you? You've become a skeleton!"

The next day Amy was taken to a doctor, diagnosed as suffering from anorexia nervosa, and referred to a psychological and nutritional counseling program. The road to recovery was not easy for the young girl. She still wanted to look like a prima ballerina and refused to believe that she was probably already thinner than most of them.

In therapy Amy had to deal with such issues as wanting to be in control and her overzealous pursuit of perfection, both in dieting and dance. At times Amy tried to trick the doctors and nutritional counselors by resorting to the same food games she used on her parents. As a result, twice when her weight plummeted to a dangerously low level she was hospitalized and forcibly fed through a tube inserted in her body.

While Amy has since made some progress, at the time

of this writing she's still in treatment. Her eating disorder
has been costly to her in a variety of ways. Due to her
lengthy hospitalizations and the physical toll anorexia nervosa took on her body, Amy was forced to stop dancing,
as well as lost a year of school. Recovering from anorexia
is often extremely difficult, especially if the problem continues for some time. Many victims require extensive therapy and Amy, who still wants to be thinner than the
thinnest ballerina, appears to be no exception.

Bulimia, also known as the binge-purge syndrome, is
another eating disorder afflicting significant numbers of
women. Unlike anorexics, bulimics generally do not starve
themselves, although they may sometimes fast for short
periods. Instead, bulimics generally eat large quantities of
high-calorie foods and avoid gaining weight through self-
induced vomiting, laxative abuse, and relentless exercise.

Bulimics are harder to spot than anorexics because they
usually maintain a normal weight for their height and
build. Yet while many bulimics manage to initially hide
their problem, they are often unable to conceal the dev-
astating toll it eventually takes on their bodies.

The continual vomiting associated with bulimia can
result in irregular heart rhythms or even heart failure and
death. In addition, some bulimics ingest drugs to induce
vomiting that destroys the heart muscle. A bulimic's esoph-
agus may tear or bleed as a result of stomach acid washing
up as she vomits. The continual vomiting simultaneously

erodes tooth enamel, increasing cavities, gum damage, and tooth discoloration. At times bulimics develop a facial puffiness known as "chipmunk cheeks," which occurs when the vomiting causes the salivary glands to swell.

Researchers recently identified a relatively new type of bulimia known as exercise bulimia. As in the standard form of the disorder afflicted individuals binge on excessive amounts of food, but instead of purging themselves through a combination of vomiting, laxatives, and exercise, they rely solely on exercise to burn off their caloric intake.

An exercise bulimic will work out for three or four hours at a time, attend an aerobics class, and then pedal five miles on an exercise bike before going to bed. Often exercise bulimics become anxious if prevented from engaging in rigorous activity, as they feel they may be putting on weight when not in motion. In some instances their need to exercise is so excessive that it interferes with their school or work responsibilities.

Ironically, at other times, an exercise bulimic who functions in other areas of her life may be praised for consistently adhering to her nearly superhuman exercise regime. Since many people avoid physically challenging workouts, the exercise bulimic is sometimes wrongly viewed as a committed fitness enthusiast rather than as suffering from a serious eating disorder. Unfortunately, exercise bulimics frequently don't think they have a problem and are especially reluctant to seek out or accept professional help.

Bulimia is thought to be extremely prevalent among models, actresses, and young girls who emulate them. According to Dr. Miriam Kaufman: "People want to be pencil thin. Models are supposed to be able to put their legs together and still have a space between their knees."[6] Among its victims was Monika Schnarre, one of Canada's best-known teen models. In 1986 this 14-year-old high school student was selected over 200,000 other girls as the Ford Modeling Agency's Super Model of the World. Shortly thereafter she signed a quarter-million-dollar contract with a prestigious New York modeling agency and appeared on the covers of over 50 magazines around the globe.

Yet maintaining the unrealistic body standard necessary for a high-fashion model was not easy for the 14-year-old who'd been transplanted from Canada to New York. She panicked when, after arriving in the United States, she began to put on weight. Although the young model stood 6'1" tall, even adding a minimal number of pounds was problematic when she had to pose in formfitting, highly styled garments.

To keep her obligations, as well as satisfy her food cravings, Schnarre began to binge and purge. When the disorder grew worse, her agent sent her home for counseling. Yet as Schnarre later recalled, "I didn't realize how sick I was." The Canadian model was fortunate—she received proper care and recovered.

Another bulimic survivor from the fashion world is Christine Alt, sister of the famous supermodel Carol Alt. After Christine graduated from high school, her family encouraged her to become a model like her sister. Although Christine managed to sign with a large New York agency, she didn't get many assignments. Feeling that she might be too heavy, the young woman began to eat less, hoping to enhance her career prospects.

At first Alt dieted sensibly, filling up on salads and vegetables while increasing her exercise level. However, when she didn't lose much weight, she continued to restrict what she ate until she barely ate anything at all. At one point she existed on seltzer water for ten days while exercising nearly three hours daily.

During this period Alt went to the modeling agency for weigh-ins. At 5'11" she was finally able to wear a size 4, but after acknowledging her accomplishment the agency merely urged her to continue. Ironically, even at her lowest weight Alt still did not get a great deal of work, since by then she often looked drawn and tired.

Though her boyfriend and parents told her to stop, Alt continued dieting. Then after having had her fill of the pressure to be as slim and sought after as her successful sister, she decided to leave New York. Alt moved to Dallas, but unfortunately, her problems with food continued. She would still try not to eat, and sometimes when she gave in to a craving, she'd force herself to throw up. Although it wasn't easy, Alt eventually overcame her eating disorder and returned to New York. She resumed modeling, only now she worked as a plus-size model and remained a comfortable size 12.

In commenting on her ordeal Christine Alt remarked: "People ask me, how can things change? It could start with parents not pressuring girls to be straight A students with Barbie doll figures. But the rest of it—most of it comes from within. And it's hard. I'm finally happy with the way I look but it took me twenty-eight years to get here."[7]

Ironically, although Christine's sister, supermodel Carol Alt, was held up as a paragon of excellence to Christine and millions of other women striving to be beautiful, the road to alluring slimness was not always easy for her. Carol hadn't initially intended to go into modeling—she was a straight A prelaw student at Hofstra University on Long Island, New York, when she caught the eye of a professional photographer who referred her to several high-powered New York City modeling agencies. She didn't call them at first, but several weeks later when she was in an adventurous mood, Alt decided to contact one and see what happened. The modeling agent she saw immediately recognized the slim, blue-eyed, dark-haired beauty's potential and told her that a wonderful career in modeling awaited her as soon as she lost 15 pounds.

Alt recalled that for her first modeling assignment an editor promised to send her on a shoot to Rome if she dropped 12 pounds. Never having been to Rome and wanting to go, Alt nearly made herself stop eating for several weeks. She'd have an apple or some celery sticks every so often, but as she only had a month to reach her goal weight, she couldn't afford many lapses.

The young model lost the weight, but unfortunately there were repercussions. While on location she had to pose in furs and heavy woolens under the hot summer sun. Weakened by the starvation regime she'd endured, Alt tried to appear upbeat and professional despite working outdoors after the temperature had soared to 97°F. However, at one point during the photo session when the photographer told her to look up, Alt collapsed instead.

As time passed, Carol Alt experimented with a variety of diets. She went on the Beverly Hills diet and ate mainly fruits, while other times she'd try to fill up on eight cups of coffee a day and have only a salad for dinner. Alt managed to remain reed slim, but before long the effects of having so little to eat each day became evident, as much of the time she felt tired, depressed, or irritable. Fortunately, she eventually saw a nutritionist and learned how to eat healthfully while remaining slender. No longer willing to live on salads and coffee, Carol Alt now allows herself to eat whatever she wants in moderation.

There have been other changes as well. Although she

still does some modeling, Alt has gone into acting. While as a model she weighed as little as 115 pounds, today Alt has abandoned this unrealistic standard and is content to maintain her weight at 127 pounds.

Numerous other supermodels who seem to have easily attained fame and financial success have actually waged desperate battles to keep their weight at the low level demanded by their profession. Among them is Kim Alexis, a tall, blue-eyed blond from Lockport, New York. Like Carol Alt, Alexis hadn't originally intended to go into modeling. As a high-school senior she competed in swimming meets and had planned on one day becoming a pharmacist. However, all that changed after the owner of the prestigious Elite modeling agency offered the young 5'10" 145-pound woman a glamorous modeling career. She could have the world in the palm of her hand if only, like Alt, the already slender young woman lost 15 pounds.

To make the grade, at one time or another Kim Alexis went on nearly every fad diet she came across. Once she even starved herself for four consecutive days. Then she tried the Atkins's diet, a weight loss plan that emphasized high-protein, low-carbohydrate food intake. Prompted by an impatient industry, she felt that she couldn't afford to adhere to any diet for very long unless it produced spectacular results. Therefore, if she wasn't able to lose ten pounds in a single week, Alexis switched to another weight loss plan. Sadly, the damage to her body caused by her bizarre eating habits soon became evident. She stopped menstruating for two years and believes that she also threw her metabolism off kilter.

Yet despite the emotional and physical sacrifices she made, Kim Alexis frequently felt as though she'd fallen short of what was expected of her. In a magazine interview Alexis noted that often she didn't feel sufficiently thin for those in charge of the photography shoot. Even if she indulged in just a plate of steamed vegetables, she might be accused of overeating, despite the meal's low calorie content. She also reported crying most of the time during the first year of her career.

Alexis sometimes felt that being humbled in this way was a sort of punishment for being beautiful, and as she grew older there were numerous self-esteem and self-image hurdles to overcome. Like many models, when she later married and had children, Alexis had to adjust to the weight gain and bloating that is part of pregnancy. The weight came off easily after her first child, but she gained 50 pounds while carrying her second baby and had a harder time losing the excess weight. Nevertheless, she claims that loving the baby more than her own self-image helped her to put vanity aside.

Like Carol Alt, these days Kim Alexis has resigned herself to weighing more than at the start of her modeling career. She's also diversified professionally to some degree. Now in her 30s, Kim Alexis hosts a weekly parenting show on cable television's Family Channel, has completed a fitness video, and serves as the celebrity spokesperson for Contempra indoor grills.

Still another extremely successful model whose weight was a dominant factor in her life is Beverly Johnson, one of the first African-American supermodels. Like Carol Alt and Kim Alexis, Johnson hadn't originally planned on going into modeling. She'd been a champion swimmer and had intended to continue her education to become an attorney. In fact, Beverly Johnson was a criminal-justice major at Northeastern University in Boston when her friends encouraged her to try modeling. At 17 Johnson walked into *Glamour* magazine's offices and was immediately offered a modeling assignment. The only stipulation was the same as it had been for Alt and Alexis—she needed to lose weight.

To satisfy the industry's demands, Johnson ate nearly nothing for extended periods, and she believes that she later developed a thyroid problem as a result of the countless crash diets she tried. Beverly Johnson achieved the required weight loss but still never felt secure in a business that placed such a high value on slenderness and physical perfection. Although she reached an enviable level of success, Johnson frequently thought that each photo she took might be her last, since she never knew when someone thinner and prettier might walk through the door.

Under the pressure to maintain an ultraslim, glamorous image, Johnson eventually fell victim to such eating disorders as anorexia nervosa and bulimia. She desperately wanted to break out of this unhealthy mode but found that she couldn't stop herself. Once, when Johnson was about 27 or 28, she visited her mother, who dragged her from the bathroom after she'd showered and forced her to look at herself in a three-way mirror. Confronted with the reality of self-starvation, she broke down in tears.

She may have been famous, but Beverly Johnson felt unhappy and out of control much of the time. Eventually a girlfriend who overheard a bulimic Johnson purging in the bathroom brought the successful model to the 12-step program Overeaters Anonymous. At first she'd hesitated to go, feeling that she wouldn't fit in with a group of obese people. But after arriving, Johnson saw that many of those attending were thin and dealing with the same feelings and problems she was. Johnson believes that she'll always have an eating disorder but hopes that with the group's help she'll be able to control it and feel better about herself.

Even though she's tried to discourage her, Beverly Johnson's 13-year-old daughter, Anansa, hopes to go into modeling as well. Johnson noted that presently the young girl is healthy, but she suspects that once her daughter is in the business, she'll be pressured into starving herself as most young models are. It's been more than 20 years since her famous mother began her career, but little has changed. Society still reveres these women as the ultimate standard of beauty, but few realize what achieving and maintaining that image can do to a woman's health and life.

Sadly, even young women who do not suffer from eating disorders rarely escape society's obsession with thinness. Four out of every five fourth-grade girls are already on diets, regardless of whether or not they need to be. The most current research further shows that a large percentage of normal women actually perceive their bodies in much the same way as those with eating disorders. Even though their figures are fine by objective standards, they'll look in the mirror and see someone who needs work.

Some women felt encouraged when a number of fashion magazines announced that ultrathin, stick-figured bodies were out while more curvaceous figures were back in style. Yet others argued that this new female ideal was perhaps even more elusive than the former. As one feminist publication described the new expectations: "Skinny muscular legs, the taut abdomen of a thirteen-year-old, and arms with the muscle definition that comes from daily work outs—that's the body we want. Looking like an underdeveloped adolescent girl is out. What's very much the rage is looking like a well-developed adolescent boy."

However, it wasn't long before the fashion pendulum swung back. The fuller-bodied, more muscular look of the 1980s and early 1990s was soon replaced by the "waif" look made famous by ultrathin supermodel Kate Moss. Moss, who's been described by a major New York newspaper as looking "like she should be tied down and intravenously fed," epitomizes the latest skin-and-bones look that women are now supposed to emulate.

To achieve this look, women must to some degree remain on a continuous, near starvation diet. As a therapist specializing in eating disorders described the predicament: "We've put this new demand on women that they be 'successful eaters.' They must look like women who are eating to be thin." It's a relentless and difficult standard to live up to, and one that young women often pay a high price for.

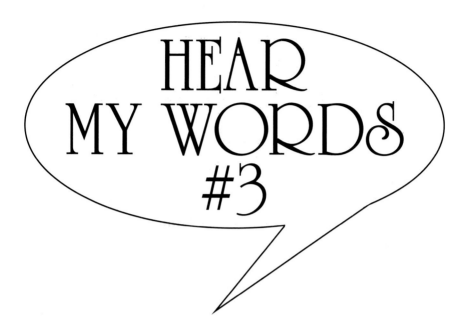

LYNN SPEAKS:

I always dreamed of being a blond. Most fairy-tale princesses were blond and the blonds in TV beer commercials were usually the best-looking girls on the screen. They were the ones the men crowded around. I realized years ago that boys go for blonds in a big way and act as if those girls are special and somehow prettier than the rest of us.

It's funny because a blond doesn't need to be that great-looking. For some reason I'll never quite understand, just having that hair color is enough. You only have to hear something like "I saw him in a convertible with a blond last night," or "He ran off with a blond," or "He nearly fell off his chair when that blond passed," and you automatically think of these girls as sexy and terrific.

But if you look at them closely, their features and bodies aren't all that different from ours. In fact, some of the better-looking girls at school have dark hair. Yet girls who really aren't gorgeous get more than their share of dates because they just happen to be blonds.

I guess sometimes I was as guilty of admiring them as everyone else. As a child, I always wanted blond dolls and treated them better than the darker ones. And when I held imaginary tea parties, I sat my blond dolls together in a special place by the window. I think I even saved the prettiest names for them, too.

As a brunette, I'd been jealous of blonds for a long time. I especially disliked the ones who grew their hair real long and had all the boys gaga over them. Tired of feeling as though I was always going to be an outsider, I finally decided to go blond. After all, what was the big deal. All that magic came out of a bottle, and I figured that with the right amount of peroxide anyone could be a blond.

Everybody tried to talk me out of it. My friends and family all said that my skin was too dark for blond hair and that I wouldn't look good in it. My mother, who had about the same coloring I did, said that she'd tried to go blond but her dark hair came out a brassy orange. She hated it and it took a long time to get back her natural color. But I felt the people around me weren't being fair. They knew me as a brunette all my life, and I thought they couldn't picture me as anything else.

I spoke to the beauty shop owner and she thought it could be done and would look okay. But when I told my mother the beautician's opinion, she just said, "What do you expect her to say—that's how she makes her living." Even though my mom never stopped telling me I'd regret it, in the end she said the decision was mine to make.

Since it was already May of my junior year in high school, I decided to do it once the term was over. I thought it would be better if I didn't see a lot of kids from school over the summer. I didn't want people to vividly remember how dark my hair had been. The summer was also good because I'd be working as a pool girl at a country club in the next town. I'd meet a bunch of new people and could try out my blondness on them before school started.

I saved up enough money to have it done just before the Fourth of July. Going blond wasn't cheap. It took all the money I'd earned over the past three months walking the neighbors' dogs plus the cash my grandparents and aunt sent me for my birthday. That meant I wouldn't be getting much of a new summer wardrobe, but I didn't care. I just wanted to be blond and have everyone make a fuss over me.

I spent nearly five hours in the beauty parlor on the

day I finally did it. I'd picked a shade of blond from a color chart, but the beautician told me that first we'd have to see how my hair took the bleach. Nobody told me that going blond could be painful, but it was. I have very sensitive skin, and the harsh dye burned my scalp, leaving painful sores. I told the beautician what was happening, but when she wanted to wash it off, I said it wasn't that bad. I'd invested too much to stop now.

I had my new life as a blond all planned out. I pictured myself being really popular and I decided to tell everybody that my folks were from Sweden. Actually, my parents were from Romania, but I was tall and I figured that with blond hair I'd look Swedish, or at least how most people pictured Swedes.

By the time I left the beauty parlor, I felt excited about my new hair color, but it was hard to get used to how I looked. My hair had come out nearly white, and you could hardly see the sores on my head unless I wore it up. The people who knew me weren't crazy about it, though. My mother thought it made me look cheap, and my brother said that I looked more like a dumb blond than a Swedish one. About the kindest comment came from our upstairs neighbor, who said, "Well, I guess it's all right if you like it."

Maybe it wasn't quite what I expected, but I kind of liked it. Somehow I'd pictured myself with silky, shining blond hair that glistened in the sunlight. But since my natural hair color was so dark, the beautician left the bleach on for a really long time. My hair came out blond, but it was also somewhat strawlike. I used conditioner on it at home, but I don't think it made much of a difference.

Things weren't bad for the first few weeks, but then my hair took a turn for the worse. With my being at the pool all day, it became brittle and began to break off. Before long I had a headful of split ends. I stopped by the beauty shop for help and was told to use a special hot oil treatment on it. But it just made my hair look greasy and flat.

Then after a while my roots started to show. Of course, it couldn't be helped. I had naturally dark hair and as it grew in, my head looked kind of horizontally striped. It had only been six or seven weeks, but the dark roots really stood out. With the rest of my hair bleached so light, the new growth seemed even darker by contrast.

I went to the beauty parlor for a touch-up, but the beautician wouldn't do my hair. By now it was extremely dry from the bleach, sun, and the pool's chlorine. She warned me that there'd be quite a bit of breakage if we did the roots. I went home determined to put up with it for a while longer. I didn't want to look even worse than I already did. But it really got to me when my brother started calling me "zebra."

I went back to the beauty shop a few days later and

insisted that the beautician do something with my hair. I figured that if I wore a bandana in the sun I'd limit the damage. I couldn't have been more wrong. I should have seen the disaster coming when a good part of my hair was left in the sink after being washed. Most of the rest broke off in small tufts during the next few days. I tried to wear a scarf around the pool whenever possible, but sometimes it was either just too hot or I had to work in the water.

My dream of looking like a Swedish blond turned out to be a painful nightmare. My social life was a mess that summer, too. I didn't feel like going anywhere or meeting new people with my hair the way it was. My boss at the country club was a really nice man, and I guess I was hoping that he wouldn't notice how bad I looked. It nearly killed me when he called me over one day and, speaking to me like a father, said, "You ought to sue the place that did your hair." He meant to be helpful, but he only made me feel worse. I guess I hadn't realized that I looked that terrible.

That's what being blond was like for me. My hair was still awful by the time school started. My mother had to buy me a wig because I refused to go to school looking as I did. It helped a bit, but the wig was heavy, and I was always afraid that it would come off or slide across my head or something. It took about a year for my hair to grow to a decent length in my natural color. It was my senior year and I resented spending it in an uncomfortable wig that looked matted whether or not I brushed it.

The blonds in the TV ads for hair color all look super. Their hair shines and they never have roots. I wanted to be like them, but I was left with what looked like clumps of white cotton candy growing on my head. Being a blond isn't always glamorous.

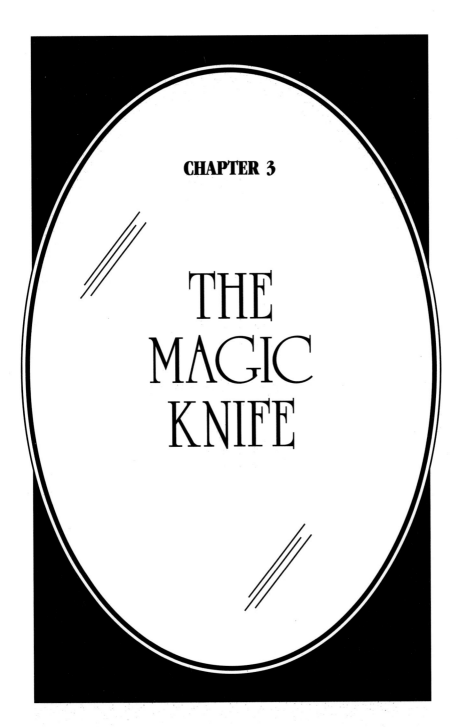

CHAPTER 3

THE
MAGIC
KNIFE

In one version of the fairy tale "The Little Mermaid," a young mermaid longs for legs so she can approach a human prince she's fallen in love with. She's granted her wish, but at a painful price— every step she takes will feel as though she is walking on broken glass. Nevertheless, the little mermaid eagerly grasps the opportunity.

Of course, that's only a story. In real life women would never endure such discomfort to make themselves more desirable to a man. Or would they?

In the 1980s the medical and advertising communities told women that the perfect look they'd dreamed of could be theirs through the "miracle" of cosmetic surgery. Women flocked to the doctors, looking for instant beauty, and the billion-dollar plastic surgery craze took off. Today many women are still routinely resorting to these procedures to revamp what they are unable to change through makeup, dieting, and rigorous exercise. While at one time plastic surgery was largely reserved for those in the entertainment industry, more recently these operations have become somewhat trendy.

Celebrities who proudly discuss their enhanced faces and figures on TV talk shows have convinced hundreds of thousands of American women that nose, ear, and chin alterations, as well as strategically placed snips and tucks, are not much more serious than applying a set of false nails. Often these adjustments are sought by women whose bodies hardly warrant change. As one Beverly Hills plastic surgeon described the situation: "Women who have perfectly nice full-sized breasts ask me if I can make them even larger. It's crazy; I tell many of them no, but I know that they can get it done somewhere else."[1]

As might be expected, women account for more than 88 percent of those desiring cosmetic surgery. Unfortunately, many seeking operations are not secure individuals who merely wish to alter a single aspect of their appearance. Instead, these females are often caught up in society's beauty trap and may be unconsciously hoping to find a speedy solution for underlying emotional problems.

As psychologist Susan Schenkel noted in a magazine interview: "You see this all the time with women's obsessions about weight. A woman will think thinness is the answer to everything that's making her unhappy in her life. Cosmetic surgery raises the issue of appearance anxiety in a more acute form because it involves a permanent alteration of the body. . . . I'd want a patient of mine to think about whether she'll feel good about herself if the surgery falls short of her expectations. Does her self-acceptance depend on a good result in the operating room?"[2]

Often such procedures are not undertaken without some degree of risk and pain. Among the most popular elective cosmetic operations in the United States today is fat vacuuming, or liposuction. Initially developed in France and introduced into the United States in 1982, the process rids the body of fat deposits that are especially resistant to diet and exercise. Liposuction is most commonly used on the face, neck, arms, breasts, abdomen, lateral thighs, inner thighs, calves, and ankles.

During liposuction the patient is usually put under general or local anesthetic. After making a small incision in the skin, the physician inserts a blunt-ended metal tube, called a cannula, and rotates the instrument to dislodge underlying fat, which is then sucked into a vacuum machine. Two to four pounds of fat may be removed at one time.

Although the notion of thin thighs in 30 minutes may

appeal to many women, liposuction is not as ideal as it sounds. While it seems quick and simple, a significant amount of pain and discomfort must be endured while healing. Patients are required to wear a tight-fitting elastic girdle or bandage over the area for up to eight weeks as well. Even though a new liposuction method known as the tumescent technique supposedly reduces the pain and recovery time involved, there is still considerable discomfort.

There are also some medical risks associated with liposuction. The vast majority of patients survive the procedure, but there have been some fatalities due to excessive blood or fluid loss, infection, or a blood or fat clot. In other instances postoperative complications included the collection of fluid beneath the skin, pulmonary embolisms, or the obstruction of blood vessels in the lungs. In cases where too much fat was removed, there may be extensive burning as well as permanent rippling of the skin.

Those best suited for liposuction are individuals near their ideal weight who have smooth, elastic skin. Ironically, the perfect liposuction candidate might be considered the person with the least need for any type of cosmetic surgery. Yet in their clamor for glamour large numbers of women have sought out the procedure to erase even the slightest body flaws.

Besides the pain and existing medical risks, liposuction is also quite costly. Fees can climb to $8,000 depending on the procedure(s) desired and are generally not covered by insurance as they are performed purely for cosmetic reasons. Nevertheless, the relentless search for physical perfection pursued by some women has caused the demand for liposuction to skyrocket.

As a clinical psychologist noted: "It's very easy for achievement-oriented people to get caught up in the quest for perfection. Women who have cosmetic surgery aren't less attractive than other women, but they are willing to go to greater lengths to change something about themselves that they don't like. How far do you go? What degree of improvement will satisfy you? These are questions every woman should ask herself before she decides to alter her appearance permanently."[3]

In recent years a number of cosmetic surgery procedures in addition to liposuction have become increasingly popular. These include face-lifts, eyelid and tummy tucks, chin implants, reshaped noses, and others. At times teenagers hoping to launch show business careers have sought plastic surgery to meet the picture-perfect standards demanded by the profession.

That was the case with one young girl who had her heart set on becoming an actress since she was three years old. In preparation she took singing and dancing lessons, but she wanted to alter her physical appearance as well. By the time she turned 14, she was determined to have her nose fixed, believing this was crucial to her industry marketability. She felt that when people looked at her, they simply saw someone who was all nose.

With her parents' consent she had the surgery performed the summer of her freshman year of high school so that she'd be completely healed when she returned to school that fall. She brought the plastic surgeon pictures of Julia Roberts and Cindy Crawford beforehand to show him how she wanted her nose to look.

Despite the painful healing process the young woman was glad she had the surgery performed. When she went back to school, she felt that boys showed a greater interest in her, and she also landed a part on a local teen TV sports program. She attributes her success to having her outward appearance match her intellect and personality.

The young woman's choice is not unusual. Teens are resorting to plastic surgery more than ever before, with 87 out of every 100 of these operations being performed on females. Apparently young women are increasingly willing to have their flesh cut and their faces and forms redesigned to meet an ideal. In a society that places such a high premium on appearance, it's not surprising.

One well-known teen who had plastic surgery prior to her 16th birthday is Soleil Moon Frye, who as a child starred in the NBC sitcom "Punky Brewster." After landing a lead role when she was seven years old, it looked as though Frye had a promising acting career ahead of her.

But when she reached her teens, the young girl believed that the way she looked would hold her back. Frye felt her breasts were disproportionately large—at 15 she stood 5'1" tall and wore a size 38DD bra. As a child, she'd become famous in the role of Punky Brewster, but now when she went out jogging boys called her "Punky Booster."

The young woman thought her large breasts made her look like a bimbo and felt that she could not even sit up straight without people looking at her as though she were a prostitute. She didn't want to just play wild or promiscuous women, but that was how male producers cast her.

To change things, Frye underwent breast reduction surgery, a six-hour operation that over 2,500 teenage girls opt for annually. During the procedure, performed at Century City Hospital in Los Angeles, the surgeon removed segments of each breast before reconstructing them so that Frye would be a size 36C. By the time he finished, nearly 4,000 stitches were required. Frye remained in the hospital while an intravenous drip of Demerol was administered to lessen the pain and discomfort.

Once the teen was off Demerol, there was still considerable soreness and bruising to contend with. She took painkillers, as well as antibiotics to kill an infection that developed in her left breast. For a time after her surgery Frye had to sleep on her back, and she was unable to comfortably lift her arms. Although the teen had hoped to be up and around in a week, it actually took about four weeks for her to heal.

Frye is pleased with the surgery and was willing to accept unavoidable trade-offs, which included not being able to one day breast-feed a child, plus having C-shaped scars under each breast and around the nipples, and a scar extending from each nipple to her rib cage.

While the actress underwent breast reduction surgery, an even greater proportion of American women have sought to enlarge their chests through breast augmentation. The type of breast enhancement most popular and at the same time most detrimental to women has been silicone breast implants. As the procedure was introduced more than 30 years ago, swarms of women have eagerly sought implants, hoping to attain Barbie doll hourglass figures. Many claim that these surgically inserted gel-filled sacs enhance both their self-esteem and overall image.

By the early 1960s more than two million women had breast implants, and about 30,000 others annually sought the procedure. In our breast-obsessed society implants were emerging as the order of the day for increasing numbers of women. "One of the exciting things about plastic surgery in Los Angeles is that it is becoming an integral part of society, just like going to the dentist or barber," a Beverly Hills cosmetic surgeon noted.[4]

Implant surgery, or breast augmentation, soon blossomed into a lucrative $50-million-a-year business, a fact that did not go unnoticed by the lobbying group, the American Society of Plastic and Reconstructive Surgeons. An early 1980s public relations campaign launched by the organization underscored the American woman's need for breast implants with a memo to the Food and Drug Administration (FDA) characterizing small breasts as an illness. It stated, "There is a substantial and enlarging body of medical information and opinion to the effect that these deformities [small breasts] are really a disease that, left uncorrected, results in a total lack of well being."[5]

To "cure" the "disease," many plastic surgeons relied on the Même implant, a silicone gel sac developed in 1982. The Même's popularity was at least partly attributable to its polyurethane foam cover, which was supposed to eliminate breast hardening, a common complication with other types of implants. Before long, women eagerly requested these newly enhanced implants, completely unaware that the foam used in them was initially developed for furniture upholstery, oil filters, and carburetors.

Through the years there were reports of problems with the Même, as well as with other implants. Yet even after rumors surfaced indicating that the health risks might be serious, some women were still willing to take that chance for the sake of beauty. Of course, at the time the risk level wasn't clear. Chemical companies manufacturing implants had grown skilled at camouflaging and even avoiding research that might interfere with their advertising campaigns to promote their products. The deception was intensified by the FDA's inadequate monitoring of breast implants.

Only later was it learned that the early animal studies on the Même were less than thorough, even though these test results were often used to assure physicians of the implant's safety. As a senior scientific advisor described the implant manufacturer's strategy: "Their approach [to testing] was rudimentary. Sorely lacking was toxicological testing for the presence of chemical by-products of the foam in the body over the short and long term. Concerns had been raised by biomaterial scientists since the early sixties about the potential of some polyurethane foams to release toxic substances, if not carcinogens. But this issue was apparently not a priority for the company."[6]

Meanwhile, women began to see more clearly that breast implants might prove hazardous to their health. Unfortunately, over the years the silicone gel envelopes often leaked into surrounding breast tissue. Some of the earlier poor-quality implant sacs even ruptured, causing their contents to spill out into the body. As the recipient's immune systems activated to combat these chemicals, inflammation and excruciating chest pain frequently resulted. In the worst instances the contaminating substances spread through their bodies, reaching the lungs, liver, and lymph nodes.

The gel's presence in the body often triggers a variety

of autoimmune disorders, including scleroderma, a condition in which the skin becomes thicker and stiffer and fibrous tissue may build up in various body organs. Silicone gel leakage can also lead to rheumatoid arthritis and a condition known as lupus erythematosus, which causes severe and persistent joint pain and widespread rashes.

Among the most frightening repercussions of silicone gel implants is the possible risk of cancer. One report by an implant manufacturer revealed that the gel sacs were proving carcinogenic in laboratory rats. In addition, an internal FDA memo indicated, "While there is no direct proof that silicone causes cancers in humans, there is considerable reason to suspect that it can do so." It also became known that implants make cancerous lumps in the breast harder to detect.

Based on this information, some women with breast implants have begun to seriously rethink their decisions. One Los Angeles woman had her implants removed after developing scleroderma and having the skin around her fingers tighten until she could barely move them. Once the implants were out, her condition significantly improved and she remarked, "I feel much better now. I wish I had realized ten years ago that how I looked was fine."[7]

Today there are countless stories of women who've suffered as a result of breast augmentation. Among the most publicized implant disasters is that of comedian-talk show host Jenny Jones. Jones, who described her father as a "breast man," had been self-conscious about having small breasts since she was a girl. Not realizing the effect it might have on their young daughter, her parents joked about her flat chest and her father suggested that she do breast enlarging exercises as well as run cold water on her chest in the shower.

As a young woman, Jones wore padded and push-up bras to make her look larger, but she still felt uncomfortable and thought that she'd never be able to wear the revealing lingerie she saw in stores. However, after a female co-worker told her about breast implants, Jones became determined to get them, even though she practically had to sell everything she owned to pay for the operation.

Jenny Jones's surgeon described a new silicone implant that tended to prevent breast hardening and added that if her breasts became hard he'd replace the implants at no cost. She agreed to try it and was operated on in May 1981. At first she felt excited about the results, but after only six months her right breast started to harden. Tired of walking around with one soft breast and the other hard as a rock, by May of the following year she'd returned to her surgeon to have the implants replaced. As promised, there was no charge for the procedure, and this time the doctor used a smaller version of the same implant, hoping for better results.

Unfortunately, both her new implants hardened within just five months. Jenny Jones went back to her surgeon in December 1983 and, after putting her under general anesthesia, he squeezed the implants to soften them. Although this was a common practice at the time, implant manufacturers later warned that excessively manipulating these devices could lead to ruptures. But in any case, the massage didn't alleviate the hardening, and on December 19, 1983, Jones underwent a third breast implant operation. Like the others, the surgery was painful and left conspicuous scars around both nipples. To Jones's disappointment her breasts soon hardened again, and after a while she lost all feeling in them.

On August 13, 1984, Jenny Jones had still another surgery—this time to try the Même implant, which was also supposed to prevent breast hardening. When she was operated on, she had no way of knowing that the Même would later be voluntarily recalled by the manufacturer due to possible cancer risks. Yet she experienced her own problems with the implants. The postoperative swelling did not subside, and just a week after the operation she underwent additional surgery to stop the internal bleeding.

In time the Même implants hardened as well, but by then the show business personality felt too discouraged to do anything about it. She tried to resign herself to what had occurred, but as she grew older and her breasts began to sag, she was left with one pointing up and the other pointing down. Jones's breasts were now badly mismatched, throwing off her cleavage and making it impossible for her to wear anything low-cut.

From 1985 to 1991 Jenny Jones saw a number of doctors to ask if anything could be done, but she was told to be grateful that this was all that had gone wrong. Then she found a physician who told her about Misti Gold, a new implant that had worked especially well with women whose other implants had hardened. Despite her past experiences Jones decided to try the new implants and on March 6, 1991, had her sixth breast operation. When a red splotch appeared on her chest in the following weeks, her doctor told her that her old implants had ruptured and that the discoloration was probably her body's reaction to the silicone left inside her. The doctor was unable to tell Jones when the spill occurred, leaving her to wonder what would happen next.

She didn't have to wait long to find out. Several months later the Misti Gold implants hardened just as all the others had. By then more information had been publicly revealed about the dangers of implants, and Jones asked her doctor to take hers out. However, she was told that if all the silicone that had seeped into her body was removed, a sizable amount of tissue would be lost and she'd probably become suicidal over the end result.

Jones decided to have the implants removed anyway. She did not become suicidal but instead feels relieved. Jenny Jones does not regret going public with her story and is glad to have had an opportunity to warn other women about breast implants. She stated: "My goal is to say to anybody who is considering implants: Don't do it. It's not worth the risk. Learn to love yourself. If I could have learned that, I wouldn't have had to suffer these eleven years of torture."[8]

As lawsuits against breast implant manufacturers mount and further research is done on the possible connection between implants and various autoimmune problems and cancer, the FDA has at least temporarily limited the availability of silicone gel implants in the United States. Yet the reaction of some young women to the ban has been disturbing. Although aware of the danger, a number of young models claim they need fuller breasts to look better and say that if necessary they'd go to Mexico for the implants.

Perhaps the excessive pressure on women to be physically alluring is best summed up by an exercise shoe commercial featuring groups of well-toned women running, jogging, and doing aerobics. The message might be one encouraging them to be healthy or enjoy sports until a song in the background states, "Stay young and beautiful if you want to be loved." Beauty is a cruel prerequisite to attach to such a universal need. Yet despite the elusiveness of loveliness, countless women risk their health and lives seeking it.

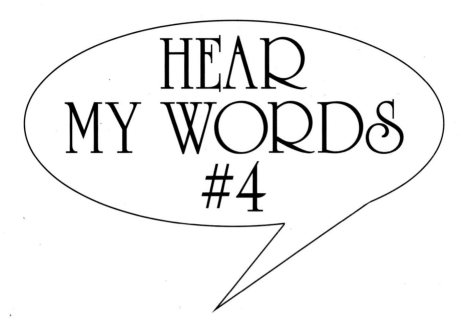

MOLLY SPEAKS:

People say that a girl with money, brains, and beauty has it all. I never had it all. My family has struggled to make ends meet since I was small and I was never any great beauty. In fact, I wasn't any kind of beauty. It's not that I'm ugly; I guess I'm just average-looking. I have the kind of face that makes people think they've met me before. I think that I look like a lot of other people.

But if I'm ordinary-looking, there's nothing ordinary about my mind. I loved school and always did well in most subjects. I graduated in the top ten of my class and did even better in college than in high school. I went to a prestigious university on scholarship and majored in geology. The geology department was small and I enjoyed working closely with the professors.

Besides earning high grades, I was well liked by my teachers and the other students. That's why when a student assistantship in the department became available I thought I might get it. These positions were difficult to come by and quite sought after. Student assistants earned good money and I needed both the experience and the cash. Since the alternative was a job in the dorm cafeteria, I was really excited about this chance. All students applying for the assistantship were invited to the department head's home. There we spent the afternoon drinking tea and speaking with the professors. And while the faculty sized up the student applicants, we sized up one another. Looking around the room, at first I felt I might be chosen. The only thing bothering me was Grace, another student who also wanted the assistantship.

Grace was the kind of girl my father called "a stunner." She was tall, and had a model's body and long, naturally curly auburn hair. To make things even more treacherous, Grace was extremely bright. I'd worked with her on several projects and been impressed.

Now we were after the same student assistantship, and as I watched her toss back her curls as she worked the room, a quiet panic swept through me. I suddenly felt that I'd probably be working in the dorm cafeteria next term.

Even though I was every bit as smart as Grace, and certainly showed as much promise in the field, I knew she'd win out.

Having everything that a male applicant needed wasn't enough if you were up against "a stunner." It wasn't fair—you didn't need breasts the size of melons or long, curly hair to analyze earthquake patterns. Nevertheless, Grace clearly had our mostly male faculty entranced.

I was right. Three weeks later I received the rejection letter. It thanked me for applying and went on to say how well qualified I was and how difficult it had been to select just one student from such a talented group. I hated what had happened, but there was nothing I could do about it. It didn't matter that I was a top student who loved geology. It obviously hadn't been enough. Regardless of how well you do academically, the beautiful woman always has the edge.

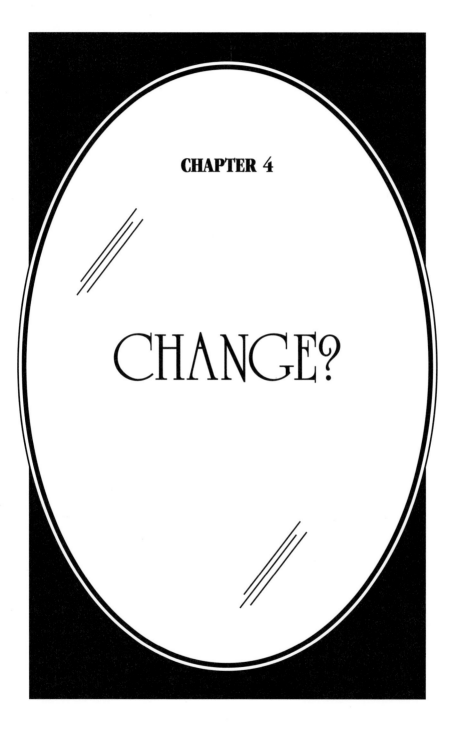

CHAPTER 4

CHANGE?

At one time a woman's life-style was often cruelly connected to her appearance. Largely deemed status trophies, beautiful women were actively pursued by successful professionals and businessmen who wanted a beautiful girlfriend or wife on their arms. Such women were often seen as dazzling human accessories that complemented a male's luxurious home, car, or job.

In the past there was no surplus of women doctors, dentists, stockbrokers, and company presidents who could afford to outfit themselves with the same trappings of achievement that were largely reserved for men. A beautiful woman was thought to be powerful in her own right—everyone's heard of ancient Greece's Helen of Troy, whose beauty was the cause of a war.

Yet in our society beauty's power is far more fleeting

than that conferred through a professional or corporate position. Unlike a medical or law degree, beauty is not an objective, tangible commodity but instead is dependent on the opinion of those around us. Such judgments are often extremely subjective and tend to fluctuate. As the saying goes, "Beauty is in the eye of the beholder," and at any given time what looks good to one person might not to another.

But even the woman regarded as exceptionally lovely by most standards often keenly knows that in our youth-oriented culture her status will fade with time. Although she might resort to expensive and even dangerous beauty treatments to retain her desirability for as long as possible, aging is inevitable. As the authors of the book *Face Value: The Politics of Beauty* concluded:

"A woman can spend her youth learning to be beautiful, and her maturity learning how it feels to be treated as beautiful, becoming used to the privileges that power confers. . . . But where possessors of other sources of power can look forward with cleverness and luck to holding on to that power to death, the beauty has to be aware that she will lose it, through no misdeed of her own, but absolutely certainly. And, like a witch's curse in a fairy tale, the loss is particularly terrifying because one never knows when it will strike . . . when your commodity may at the very moment you need to call on it already have vanished."[1]

However, with the rise of the mid-1960s women's movement, many hoped that women could now pursue prominent positions rather than merely serve as ornaments for men who did. American women began protesting their decorative status and demanded to be treated as equals. There were marches, rallies, manifestos, and lawsuits designed to redefine women as worthy of comparable treatment in all walks of life.

Change was clearly in the air when in 1966 feminists demonstrated to protest the firing of airline stewardesses who'd turned 32, and the following year the Equal Employment Opportunity Commission initiated hearings on sex discrimination.

By the start of the next decade early feminist demands had been somewhat incorporated into law. The Equal Employment Opportunity Act of 1972 promised to break down the barriers that kept women out of high-level positions, and by 1978 a fourth of the students graduating with accounting degrees were females. More than ever before it looked as though a woman's appearance might finally become secondary to her mind and talent, as large numbers of American women stepped forward to take their rightful place in the work world. As feminist Naomi Wolf described in her book *The Beauty Myth: How Images of Beauty Are Used against Women:*

"In the United States between 1960 and 1990, the number of women lawyers and judges rose from 7,500 to

180,000; women doctors from 15,672 to 108,200; women engineers from 7,404 to 174,000. In the past fifteen years the number of women in local elected office tripled to 18,000. Today in the United States women will fill 50 percent of entry-level management positions, 25 percent of middle management, comprise half the graduating accountants, one-third of the M.B.A.'s, half of graduating lawyers, and a fourth of doctors, and half the officers and managers in the fifty largest commercial banks. Sixty percent of women officers in *Fortune's* survey of top companies average $117,000 a year."[2]

It appeared as if women had overcome a major hurdle, but a closer look at the situation revealed that things might not be as rosy as they seemed. While the new women professionals and corporate executives were expected to be as competent as their male counterparts, in many instances they continued to face an unstated job requirement. Unfortunately, regardless of their ability in either the operating room or boardroom, women were still supposed to look good.

The dual standard of appearance for men and women was perhaps best illustrated through the fate of Christine Craft, the 36-year-old television news anchor who was fired by Metromedia in Kansas City because she was "too old, too unattractive, and not deferential to men." What happened to Christine Craft was not unusual. Many female news anchors feel that "looking 40" often marks the end of their careers, while men in their 50s and 60s doing the same job tend to be viewed as distinguished and knowledgeable.

Even prior to the Craft incident other women at the studio had been forced to leave their positions due to what was described as the network's "fanatical obsession" with how they looked. These incidents were repeated across the country as network recruiters rated a woman's physical appearance as even more important than her news delivery skills. Before her dismissal Craft had endured a series of company-ordered make-overs as well as time-consuming fittings for clothes she was made to purchase but would not have chosen for herself. The network's male anchors weren't required to go through these rigors, but because she was a woman, beauty became an essential aspect of Craft's job.

There was speculation that Craft's employers had not counted on her challenging her job loss. As appearance is so societally tied to being female, it seemed doubtful that a television personality would publicly announce that she was thought to be too ugly to effectively function at work. Such deep-cutting personal humiliations generally remain private. However, Metromedia underestimated Craft—she sued her ex-employers in court, charging sex discrimination. Nevertheless, she was not left unscathed by the criticism leveled at her. Craft described its effect as follows:

"Though I may have dismissed intellectually that statement that I was too unattractive, nonetheless in the core of my psyche I felt that something about my face was difficult, if not monstrous to behold. It's hard to be even mildly flirtatious when you're troubled by such a crippling point of view."[3]

Regrettably, in the end Christine Craft lost her legal battle. Although two juries found in her favor, a male judge later overturned their verdicts. Having dared to go to court, Craft subsequently found herself unable to secure other positions in her field. When another woman reporter was asked how what happened affected women in broadcast journalism, she replied: "There are thousands of Christine Crafts. We keep silent. Who can survive a blacklist?" Christine Craft's experience underscored to women that regardless of how well they hone their skills, they still must be concerned with being pretty.

Sadly, this reality extends far beyond the news and entertainment worlds. Christine Craft's story isn't all that different from that of the teenage girl who's thrown off the cheerleading squad for putting on five pounds. It's the same fear that sometimes motivates girls to go to extremes in altering their appearance, whether it's to get asked to the prom or pursue a modeling career.

The situation becomes increasingly serious when young women educationally and entrepreneurially advance only to find that they still haven't escaped the pervasive beauty trap. In the past females frequently coped with the problem through plastic surgery, stringent dieting, and products that promised to remove cellulite. But today more women are fighting back in positive ways, refusing to pay homage to a standard that limits their potential as human beings.

This was evident in the late 1980s class action suit filed against American Airlines by 13,500 flight attendants who charged their employer with sex and age discrimination. The issue arose as a result of the stringent weight requirements still maintained by the airline. The women argued that the company's requirements were unrealistic since they ignored the natural weight gain that comes with age, and discriminatory since weight standards differed for men and women.

A case in point was that of flight attendant Andrea Strauss, who'd worked for the airline for 23 years and had amassed an assortment of impressive accolades from both passengers and fellow crew members. These included complimentary letters from customers and two nominations from the staff for the "Someone Special in the Air" designation. Yet despite her exemplary performance and length of service, Strauss found herself in trouble with the airline.

Since the flight attendant was 5'6" tall, the most regulations permitted her to weigh was 133 pounds, a weight she'd maintained 20 years previously as a young woman. However, now that she wore a size 14 uniform, she no longer presented the model image her employer sought.

Many in the industry had hoped things had improved for flight attendants over the last 30 years following a number of lengthy feminist-motivated antidiscrimination court battles based on the 1964 Civil Rights Act. Since that time many airlines had either partially or totally disregarded their weight, age, and marital status restrictions. For example, in 1987, following a lawsuit, Pan Am dropped its policy of making women adhere to the weight range given for people with medium frames while male employees were permitted to use the large frame weight ranges indicated on the chart.

But Strauss's employer clung to the company's old regulations, which meant enforcing one of the strictest standards in the industry. The resulting negative repercussions on Andrea Strauss's life were unavoidable. If a supervisor suspected that a staff member was in violation of the weight requirement, she might insist that the flight attendant step on the scale for a weigh-in. If the staff member in question exceeded the standard, the employee would be placed on "weight check" and required to either lose one and a half pounds a week or be suspended without pay. If the individual did not lose the weight while suspended, she faced dismissal.

Despite her outstanding job performance, Andrea Strauss had frequently been put on weight checks, as well as suspended over a dozen times for weighing too much.

As Strauss described her ordeal: "The last time, my supervisor got on the airplane and there were probably ten passengers and the rest of the crew still on board and she said right in front of God and everybody, 'Honey, I'm going to need a weight slip from you.' Oh, yeah, it was very embarrassing."[4]

Colleen Brenner, the union's vice president, noted that although only two women were recently fired over weight concerns, "there are hundreds like Andrea who were monitored at any given time."[5] Frequently they were so humiliated that they didn't say anything to the union about what was happening to them until it was too late. Ashamed of their deviation from the slim, trim image expected of them, they often felt uncomfortable appealing to an outside source for assistance.

However, the union believes that women were actually being singled out for this type of discrimination, citing that weight requirements were generally not strictly enforced when it came to other classes of employees. "Even pilots, the front runners as far as representing the company, didn't have weight standards," Brenner added.[6] Instead, they were merely required to undergo an annual Federal Aviation Administration physical.

The unrealistic and in some cases unattainable weight requirements imposed by the company on women resulted in a host of emotional, health, and financial problems for many employees. A union-conducted survey of female staff members revealed that a high percentage of these women had suffered from eating disorders such as anorexia nervosa and bulimia and at times became addicted to diet pills. In other instances female employees had also undergone liposuction as well as sought psychiatric counseling for severe anxiety and paranoia. Ironically, while the company sponsored a drug and alcohol rehabilitation program, there were no comparable resources for employees with eating disorders. The company also did not pay for medically supervised weight reduction plans.

At times competent flight attendants who were fired because they gained weight suffered serious financial setbacks. One such woman had been suspended for about 18 months prior to her dismissal in 1988. She described the monetary consequences as follows: "I was making $2,400 a month, and went to working part-time in a retail store making $4.50 an hour. It was hard to get over that disaster financially."[7]

The weight restrictions were often more difficult for the older flight attendants to meet, since a person's metabolism tends to slow down with age and fewer calories are burned. Some staff members suspect that the company refused to relinquish the weight standards in order to force older, higher-paid flight attendants to retire so they could recruit younger, less costly labor.

Whatever the reasons behind the company's actions, female flight attendants rebelled. Anxious to make the public aware of their problem and enlist support, these women appeared on national TV talk shows, hired a public relations consultant to further the cause, and boldly posted the following demand on billboards: WEIGH MY JOB PERFORMANCE, NOT MY BODY.

This trend of women refusing to be treated as objects has caused some to say that a third wave of feminism may be coming into its own. The key vital signs are all around us. One important indicator might be the emergence of Hillary Rodham Clinton as the nation's first lady, since our first ladies often reflect the country's mood and tempo. Jacqueline Kennedy was a fashionable hostess whose emphasis on glamour, style, and demureness epitomized the role of a "wife" as the ultimate accessory to the successful man. Nancy Reagan has sometimes been said to symbolize the high-living, extravagant eighties.

But Hillary Rodham Clinton has carved out a unique role for herself as first lady and presents an intriguing glance at the direction in which American women may be heading. Clinton has long been perceived as an energetic powerhouse of talent. As an undergraduate at Wellesley College, she was elected student body president, and later her memorable speech as the first student commencement speaker was published in *Time* magazine.

From there the promising young student went on to Yale Law School, where she served as editor of the highly regarded *Yale Law Review*, as well as graduated at the top of her class. As her career advanced, she became an active partner in a prominent law firm and was rated one of the top 100 lawyers in America. While a corporate attorney, she was reported to earn more than $203,000 a year, as opposed to her husband's annual salary of $34,527 as Arkansas's governor.

Hillary Rodham Clinton's independence and drive became nationally evident following her husband's 1992 ascendancy to the presidency. While previous first ladies set up their offices in the east wing of the White House, Hillary Rodham Clinton established her working area in the west wing, where the president's staff is headquartered and much of the important decision making is done. She further broke precedent by being the first presidential wife to visit Capitol Hill and huddle with Democratic senators on nationally relevant issues. Early on in his term her husband appointed her to head the task force on health care reform. That meant that once again she'd be charting new territory as the first presidential wife to ever be assigned an official role in formulating domestic policy.

Yet perhaps even more remarkable than the first lady's achievements is the visible pride her husband takes in her ability. On numerous occasions President Clinton has publicly praised her leadership qualities and the way she skillfully tackles and resolves complex problems. Much of the country seems to agree with his assessment of her. An NBC News/ *Wall Street Journal* poll indicated that 74 percent of Americans view the first lady as a positive role model. Could Hillary Rodham Clinton's inroads at our nation's capital be representative of an upcoming era in which women may be valued for their minds without regard to their bra size or legs?

In some ways the country is ripe for a change. By the early 1990s more females than males were graduating from college and more women than men went into business for themselves. Yet in the past even well-credentialed women had to contend with the double standard of needing both brains and beauty to be considered desirable.

Ironically, the difference today may be that men are beginning to highly value smart women for largely economic reasons. In a society in which it has become difficult for a family to exist on a single income, wives frequently have had to help their husbands support their life-style. As the days when men bought everything, including ornamental wives, disappear, women with greater earning potential may become increasingly desirable. While once men bragged about their wives' or girlfriends' figures, now they often take tremendous pride in her doctorate or medical degree. The optimistic outcome is that girls who formerly hid their intelligence to make boys feel smarter may find that doing well at a prestigious college is actually a social advantage.

However, it's unrealistic to think that the age-old power battle between the sexes has been resolved. Not all males are willing to readily accept this change in our social order. Hillary Rodham Clinton, for one, has endured a great deal of criticism for both being intelligent and asserting herself. During the 1992 presidential race the Republican party characterized her as the embodiment of all that's wrong with family values, career mothers, and forward thinking women. Outspoken radio talk show host Rush Limbaugh plays a bit of the tune "Hail to the Chief" whenever he mentions the first lady's name. Hillary Rodham Clinton has also been featured on the cover of a popular magazine outfitted as a dominatrix. In some parts of the country radio stations even play an unflattering song about the first lady sung to the tune of Helen Reddy's feminist anthem "I Am Woman." It begins as follows: "I am Hillary, hear me roar, I'm more important than Al Gore."

Admittedly, Hillary Rodham Clinton has shown perseverance in remaining her own person despite the criticism of those who would hem her in. Effectively serving as a role model for modern women on the cutting edge of their generation, she noted, "The work that I have done as a professional, a public advocate, has been aimed . . . to assure that women can make the choices . . . whether it's full-time career, full-time motherhood, or some combination."[8]

Today younger women involved in what could be a budding reemergence of feminism are working for the chance to grow and be valued as full human beings. An

important part of this effort entails breaking free of the
beauty trap and leaving the concept of women as attractive trinkets behind them. There's strength in numbers,
and the number of women already in higher education is
on the rise. While in 1961 women comprised only 37 percent of the student body, by 1993 more than half of the
college students in America were women, and on numerous campuses they've set out to make their presence felt
in a way that challenges the status quo.

Large numbers of these women grew up in single-
parent households headed by women or had mothers
who worked outside the home. Seeing the significant
women in their lives effectively function independently,
they want more out of college than many women did a
generation ago. According to one such student who
recently graduated from a Boston-area college: "Our
expectations are a lot higher. We're coming to school
expecting to be treated like human beings and we're
shocked when we're not."[9]

To improve the situation, campus organizations
formed and led by women have taken on meaningful
issues and fought for change. The gains they've already
achieved are evident on numerous campuses. At Princeton, following protest demonstrations and legal action,
women were finally permitted to join the formerly all-
male eating clubs at the school. Male fraternities on the
campuses of Middlebury, Wesleyan, Bowdoin, Trinity, and

Pomona colleges have gone coed as the result of pressure from women's groups as well.

Women at Brown University, tired of the school's lax approach to dealing with date rape offenders, took matters into their own hands. These students listed the guilty parties' names on a stall door in a campus lavatory. The university administration, which initially referred to the women as the "Magic Marker terrorists," had the list removed by the janitorial staff only to find it back up again.

The women's ongoing protest led to a heated debate on campus that resulted in school officials sponsoring an open forum on the problem of sexual assault at the institution. In preparation the women drew up a list of vital demands that, among others, included instituting a sexual assault policy, provisions for filing these complaints, hiring a dean for women's issues, and requiring perpetrators to appear before a disciplinary board.

Convinced that the administration was not going to take them seriously, the women turned the forum into a protest rally. Hundreds attending wore red, and many carried signs bearing unsympathetic quotes from school administrators who were obviously not ready to make the necessary changes. However, after the national media picked up on the women's plight, the institution became increasingly responsive and granted most of the students' demands.

Similar actions were initiated and carried out by women at a number of other schools. After hearing about two campus rapes Antioch University students formed a group they named Womyn of Antioch. The group developed a policy for handling sexual offenses on campus that was later instituted by school officials.

Women at Duke University wanted male students to have a taste of what it's like for women who've been caught off guard at night and sexually accosted. An activist group known as the Date Rape and Sexual Assault Task Force surprised campus males they found walking alone after dark by jumping out and tagging them with bright orange stickers that read "Gotcha." They also provided the men with printed information on rape and sexual assault.

These and other student actions have led to genuine change. Today there are substantially more rape awareness centers at colleges across America than ever before, and Congress also passed the College Security Act, requiring colleges and universities to make their crime statistics available to the public. In the past many schools tended to cover up campus assaults against women to prevent negative publicity from possibly lowering future enrollment.

As one student activist described the change in academic environments: "We have a vocabulary now to talk about these issues in a political way. We have the resources and ability to look at things like sexual assault as societal problems, not just individual problems."[10]

Still another issue campus feminists have taken on is that of sexual harassment. The young women stress that this can be especially disconcerting when it involves faculty members, since it encompasses both male dominance over women and a professor's abuse of power over a student. In the past many women quietly dealt with the problem on their own. Often thinking that they were in some way responsible for their teacher's advances, they'd drop the course, transfer to another school, or at times feel forced to give in to their teacher's sexual demands.

Even though studies indicate that over a quarter of all college females have been sexually harassed for many years, institutions of higher learning largely ignored the problem. If the student was over 18 years of age, some even felt that relationships between consenting adults did not concern the administration.

However, psychologist Shirley Feldman-Summers, who has treated victims of sexual harassment, believes that the issue of consent becomes particularly hazy in teacher-student interactions. As Dr. Feldman-Summers asks: "If there is an unequal power relationship, can there really be free consent? And if it's consentual, can the professor be fair in his treatment of her, and can the other students [in the class] be sure they're being fairly evaluated?"[11] Following the 1986 Supreme Court ruling making employers liable for acts of sexual harassment committed by their staffs, some administrations officially registered their disapproval in personnel manuals and at faculty meetings but generally still took little or no action in these situations.

However, an increased level of campus consciousness regarding this offense and subsequent changes in school policies and actions have resulted from the persistent efforts of feminist activist groups. Women demanding reforms at colleges and universities throughout the country either filed lawsuits or threatened to take harassers to court. Princeton University feminists warned administration officials that they'd picket and boycott the classes of a professor about to be reinstated after having been suspended for sexual harassment.

In Massachusetts students who felt their school's sexual harassment policy was weak resorted to guerrilla theater tactics to publicize their cause. A group of 16 students called the Defense Guard separately circled several staff members known to have sexually harassed young women and loudly chanted their complaint.

In some instances female high-school students have also acted to deter sexual harassment. In suburban Atlanta a young woman coerced into having sex with her teacher for more than 15 months eventually sued him in court. Wanting to protect her classmates, the girl decided to take action after learning that the same teacher was making advances at other students. She initially reported what had occurred to both a teacher and a school guidance counselor. But when the guidance counselor related her accusations to the principal, he did not believe her.

Fortunately, the girl's family stood firmly behind her, since it was difficult for her to continue at that school after that. School officials never thoroughly investigated her charges of sexual harassment, and one faculty member even urged her to drop the matter before she embarrassed herself further.

But the teenager knew that what happened to her was wrong and she did not back down. Instead, she filed a complaint with the Office of Civil Rights, which, following an investigation, determined that her rights had been violated. The office cited that the sexual harassment she'd endured had interfered with her ability to receive an equal opportunity education. At that point the young woman's attorney launched a civil suit for damages in the federal district court in Atlanta.

At first the girl and her family were disappointed when the judge refused to hear the case on the grounds that students, unlike employees, could not sue for damages. The situation didn't look any better after Georgia's appeals court upheld the district court's ruling. However, the sexually harassed teen refused to give up. Her lawyer later argued her case before the Supreme Court, which in a unanimous decision determined that she had the right to sue.

Numerous high-school girls have also taken steps to

stop sexual harassment by their male classmates. At many schools they have pushed for measures to end inappropriate, sexually explicit conduct aimed at female students. While written policies prohibiting sexual harassment are now becoming more commonplace, one of the pioneering efforts in this realm was Amherst (Massachusetts) Regional High School's sexual harassment policy.

This document, included in the school's 1990 student handbook, was thought to be especially relevant since it precisely specified which behaviors were considered offensive as well as the consequences offenders would face. The unacceptable behaviors included "staring or leering with sexual overtones, spreading sexual gossip, and pressure for sexual activity," while the consequences ranged from apologizing to the victim to a "recommendation for expulsion from school" or a "referral to police."

High-school teens fighting sexual harassment have also composed carefully drafted warning letters to the people harassing them, a technique initially developed by the *Harvard Business Review* and later adapted for student use by a New England educational consultant. Frequently written with the help of a parent, teacher, or guidance counselor, this correspondence carefully details what the victim perceives as the problem, how it's affecting her, and the measures she intends to take if the abuse doesn't immediately stop.

In recent years young feminists have tackled other

important issues as well. Female college students have protested the blatant lack of women writers studied in university-level English courses. "In my literature class we only study male writers," one young woman noted. "I looked at the list like I was surprised and asked the teacher what women writers we were going to study. . . . He looked blank. I mentioned some names. He said he'd never read them. . . . This was a complete shock to the department that we were raising these issues [because] silent obedience is a strong part of the culture for women here."[12]

In response to petitions and protests some schools have revamped their curricula to reflect women writers and artists. In numerous instances departments and classes on women's studies have been organized to pass on feminist history and theory. In addition, more than ever before, women have secured professorships at colleges and universities and a few have even become presidents of institutions of higher learning.

Young feminists hoping to change the way women are viewed and treated in our society ask what would happen if little girls were raised as little boys are—to love and accept themselves for their unique accomplishments. Would pressure to conform to a rigid and unrealistic measure of female beauty fall by the wayside if the vast majority of women simply ignored it? It may be difficult to picture things that way, but at one time slavery was legal and women weren't even allowed to vote.

As one young woman described her stance on the issue: "I was introduced to feminism by my older sisters who were activists in college. They would come home on breaks and start talking about it and I would listen. At about age 11, I started reading a lot of feminist books, and I began to understand these texts as truths, especially when discriminatory situations manifested themselves in my fifth- and sixth-grade world. Even in elementary school, the sexism was obvious to me, and I thought, 'I need to be part of the feminist movement.'"[13]

Whether or not women ultimately reject the beauty trap may largely depend on what young women want for themselves and their daughters. Perhaps the women of tomorrow will find the strength to finally free themselves.

ENDNOTES

Chapter 1
1. Abigail Heyman, *Growing Up Female: A Personal Photojournal* (New York: Holt, Rinehart and Winston, 1974), unpaged.
2. Gretchen Morgenson, "Barbie Does Budapest," *Forbes,* January 7, 1991, 66.
3. Sally Stich, "All Dolled Up," *New Choices,* April 1991, 93.
4. Michelle Green, "As a Tiny Plastic Star Turns 30, the Real Barbie and Ken Reflect on Their Life in the Shadow of the Dolls," *People Weekly,* March 6, 1989, 189.
5. Ibid.
6. Sally Stich, "All Dolled Up," 93.
7. Joanna Elm, "It Takes a Ton of Money to Make It to Atlantic City—And That's Not All," *TV Guide,* September 8, 1990, 14.
8. Dalma Heyn, "Beyond the Valley of the Beautiful Dolls," *Mademoiselle,* November 1987, 182.
9. Lisa de Paulo, "The Ten Biggest Myths about the Miss America Pageant," *TV Guide,* September 6, 1986, 4.

Chapter 2
1. Elissa Melamed, *Mirror, Mirror: The Terror of Not Being Young* (New York: Linden Press, 1983), 157.
2. Marcia Millman, *Such a Pretty Face: Being Fat in America* (New York: W. W. Norton & Company, 1980), 106.
3. Brad Hamilton, "Fat's No Fun," *New York Post,* April 29, 1983.

4. "What Causes Bulimia?" *USA Today,* February 1988.
5. Janis Graham, "The Great Diet Docs," *Harper's Bazaar,* July 1991, 10.
6. D'arcy Jenish, "A Tragic Obsession," *Maclean's,* October 9, 1989, 52.
7. Christine Alt, "Viewpoint," *Glamour,* March 1992, 150.

Chapter 3
1. Steven Finlay, "Buying the Perfect Body," *U.S. News & World Report,* May 1, 1989, 69.
2. Susan Jacoby, "The Cosmetic Surgery Boom," *Glamour,* March 1988, 348.
3. Ibid., 350.
4. D'arcy Jenish, "Beauty and the Breast," *Maclean's,* March 9, 1992, 38.
5. Nicholas Regush, "Toxic Breasts," *Mother Jones,* January/February 1992, 26.
6. Ibid.
7. Andrew Purvis, "A Strike against Silicone," *Time,* January 20, 1992, 41.
8. Giovanna Breu, "Body of Evidence," *People Weekly,* March 2, 1992, 62.

Chapter 4

1. Robin Tolmach Lakoff and Raquel L. Scherr, *Face Value: The Politics of Beauty* (Boston: Routledge & Kegan, 1984), 20.
2. Naomi Wolf, *The Beauty Myth: How Images of Beauty Are Used against Women* (New York: William Morrow, 1991), 25.
3. Ibid., 36.
4. Mary Suh, "A Future up in the Air," *Ms.,* September 1989, 93.
5. Ibid.
6. Ibid.
7. Ibid.
8. Margaret Carlsen, "All Eyes on Hillary," *Time,* September 14, 1992, 30.
9. Karen Houppert, "Wildflowers among the Ivory: New Campus Radicals," *Ms.,* September/October 1991, 32.
10. Ibid., 52.
11. Ibid., 57.
12. Ibid., 58.
13. "Speak for Themselves," *Ms.,* March/April 1991, 29.

FOR FURTHER READING

Cohen, Marcia. *The Sisterhood: The True Story of Women Who Changed the World.* New York: Simon & Schuster, 1988.

Davis, Flora. *Moving the Mountain: The Women's Movement in America since 1960.* New York: Simon & Schuster, 1991.

Faludi, Susan. *Backlash: The Undeclared War against American Women.* New York: Crown, 1991.

Gay, Kathlyn. *Breast Implants: Making Safe Choices.* New York: New Discovery Books, 1993.

Jackson, Donna. *How to Make the World a Better Place for Women—In 5 Minutes a Day.* New York: Hyperion, 1992.

Lakoff, Robin Tolmach, and Raquel L. Scherr. *Face Value: The Politics of Beauty.* Boston: Routledge & Kegan, 1984.

Linden-Ward, Blanche, and Carol Hurd Green. *American Women in the 1960s: Changing the Future.* New York: Twayne, 1992.

Melamed, Elissa. *Mirror, Mirror: The Terror of Not Being Young.* New York: Linden Press, 1983.

Millman, Marcia. *Such a Pretty Face: Being Fat in America.* New York: W. W. Norton & Company, 1980.

Morgan, Robin. *The World of a Woman.* New York: W. W. Norton & Company, 1992.

Wharton, Mandy. *Rights of Women.* New York: Franklin Watts, 1989.

Wolf, Naomi. *The Beauty Myth: How Images of Beauty Are Used against Women.* New York: William Morrow, 1991.

ORGANIZATIONS CONCERNED ABOUT THE STATUS OF WOMEN

All Nations Women's League
PO Box 428
Jackson Heights, Queens, NY 11372

American Council for Career Women
PO Box 50825
New Orleans, LA 70150

Black Women's Network
PO Box 12072
Milwaukee, WI 53212

Capitol Hill Women's Political Caucus
Longworth House Office Building
PO Box 599
Washington, DC 20515

Center for the American Woman and Politics
Eagleton Institute of Politics
Rutgers University
New Brunswick, NJ 08901

Center for Women Policy Studies
2000 P Street NW, Suite 508
Washington, DC 20036

Commission for Women's Equality
c/o American Jewish Congress
15 East 84 Street
New York, NY 10028

Committee on South Asian Women
Texas A & M University
Department of Psychology
College Station, TX 77843

Congressional Caucus for Women's Issues
2471 Rayburn House Office Building
Washington, DC 20515

Equity Policy Center
2000 P Street NW, Suite 508
Washington, DC 20036

Federation of Organizations for Professional Women
2001 S Street NW, Suite 500
Washington, DC 20009

Feminist Center for Human Growth and Development
300 East 75 Street, Suite 26D
New York, NY 10021

Inter-American Commission of Women
c/o Organization of American States
1889 F Street NW, Room 880
Washington, DC 20006

Justice for Women
100 Witherspoon Street, Room 4608A
Louisville, KY 40202

Legal Advocates for Women
320 Clement
San Francisco, CA 94118

Mexican American Women's National Association
1030 15 Street NW, Suite 468
Washington, DC 20005

Ms. Foundation for Women
141 Fifth Avenue, Suite 6S
New York, NY 10010

National Association of Commissions for Women
YWCA Building, Sixth Floor
624 9 Street NW
Washington, DC 20001

National Association of Cuban-American Women of the U.S.A.
2119 South Webster
Fort Wayne, IN 46802

National Conference of Puerto Rican Women
5 Thomas Circle NW
Washington, DC 20005

National Council for Research on Women
Sara Delano Roosevelt Memorial House
530 Broadway, Tenth Floor
New York, NY 10012

National Council of Career Women
3202 Gemstone Court
Oakton, VA 22124

National Council of Women of the United States
777 United Nations Plaza
New York, NY 10017

National Organization for Women
1000 16 Street NW, Suite 700
Washington, DC 20036

National Women's Party
Sewall-Belmont House
144 Constitution Avenue NE
Washington, DC 20002

National Women's Political Caucus
1275 K Street NW, Suite 750
Washington, DC 20005

9 to 5, National Association of Working Women
614 Superior Avenue NW, Room 852
Cleveland, OH 44113

Organization of Chinese American Women
1300 N Street NW, Suite 100
Washington, DC 20005

Women Against Pornography
PO Box 845, Times Square Station
New York, NY 10036

Women's Action Alliance
370 Lexington Avenue, Suite 603
New York, NY 10017

Women's Law Project
125 South Ninth Street, Suite 401
Philadelphia, PA 19107

Women's Legal Defense Fund
1875 Connecticut Avenue NW, Suite 710
Washington, DC 20009

Women's Research and Education Institute
1700 18 Street NW, Suite 400
Washington, DC 20009

Women's Rights Project
c/o American Civil Liberties Union
132 West 43 Street
New York, NY 10036

INDEX

A

advertising media, 29, 40, 46, 63, 65, 71, 74, 75, 88
Alexis, Kim, 59-61
Alt, Carol, 56, 57-59
Alt, Christine, 56-57
American Airlines, 100
American Association of University Women, 25
American Society of Plastic and Reconstructive Surgeons, 82
Anderson, Wayne, 46

B

Barbie dolls, 23-27, 41, 57, 81
Beauty Myth: How Images of Beauty Are Used against Women, The, 96
beauty pageants, 26-31, 34
   Little Miss of America, 26, 28, 34
   Miss America, 9, 26, 28-34
   Miss Teenage America, 26, 34
   Miss Universe, 9, 34
blonds, 65-71
breast surgery and implants, 75, 80-88
Brenner, Colleen, 102

C

Cabbage Patch babies, 41
children, 18-26, 63

Clinton, Hillary Rodham, 104-107
Clinton, President Bill, 105
College Security Act, 110
cosmetic surgery, 11, 17, 28, 30, 75-88, 100
Craft, Christine, 97-99

D

dieting, 17, 35, 36, 41, 47, 50-52, 56, 58, 59, 61, 63, 64, 75, 100, 103

E

eating disorders, 11, 47, 53, 54, 57, 62-64, 103
   anorexia nervosa, 47, 48, 52, 53, 62, 103
   bulimia, 47, 53-55, 62, 103
Elite modeling agency, 59
Equal Employment Opportunity Act of 1972, 96
exercise, 29, 41, 51, 53, 54, 56, 75, 88

F

Face Value: The Politics of Beauty, 95
fairy tales, 20-23, 26, 31, 65, 74, 95
Feldman-Summers, Shirley, 111

feminists, 25, 96, 101, 107,
    110, 112, 114-116
Food and Drug Administration
    (FDA), 82-84, 88
Ford Modeling Agency's Super
    Model of the World, 55
Frye, Soleil Moon, 79-81

H
Handler, Ken, 25
Hassan, Abu, 34

J
Johnson, Beverly, 61-63
Jones, Jenny, 84-88

K
Kaufman, Dr. Miriam, 55
Kennedy, Jacqueline, 104

L
Lambert, Leslie, 42-46
Limbaugh, Rush, 107
liposuction, 76-78, 103

M
makeup, 27, 29, 30, 75
Mattel, 24, 25
Metromedia, 97, 98
Mickley, Dr. Diane, 47
models, 55-62, 99, 101
Motz, Marilyn, 24
Munoz, Amparo, 34

P
Pan Am airlines, 101
professional women, 94-97,
    106, 115

R
Reagan, Nancy, 104
Reverly, Susan, 25
Rizk, Georgina, 34
role models, 24, 106, 107
Rubens, 41

S
Sapps, Carolyn Suzanne, 32-33
Schenkel, Susan, 76
Schnarre, Monika, 55-56
self-image, 60, 81
sexual assault and harrassment,
    109-114
sexual discrimination, 96-100,
    108
Strauss, Andrea, 100-102

T
Tautkas, Richard, 42
teenagers, 10, 26, 43, 55,
    78-80, 99, 113, 114

W
weight and acceptance, 30,
    35-38, 40-63, 76, 77,
    100-103
Winfrey, Oprah, 36, 37
Wolf, Naomi, 96

ABOUT THE AUTHOR

Popular author Elaine Landau worked as a newspaper reporter, an editor, and a youth services librarian before becoming a full-time writer. She has written more than 55 nonfiction books for young people, including *Woman, Woman!: Feminism in America* and *Why Are They Starving Themselves: Understanding Anorexia Nervosa and Bulimia.*

Ms. Landau, who has a bachelor's degree in English and journalism from New York University and a master's degree in library and information science from Pratt Institute, now lives in New Jersey.